The Guide to
NATURAL
THERAPIES

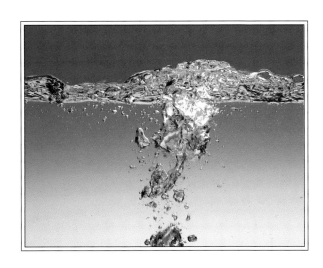

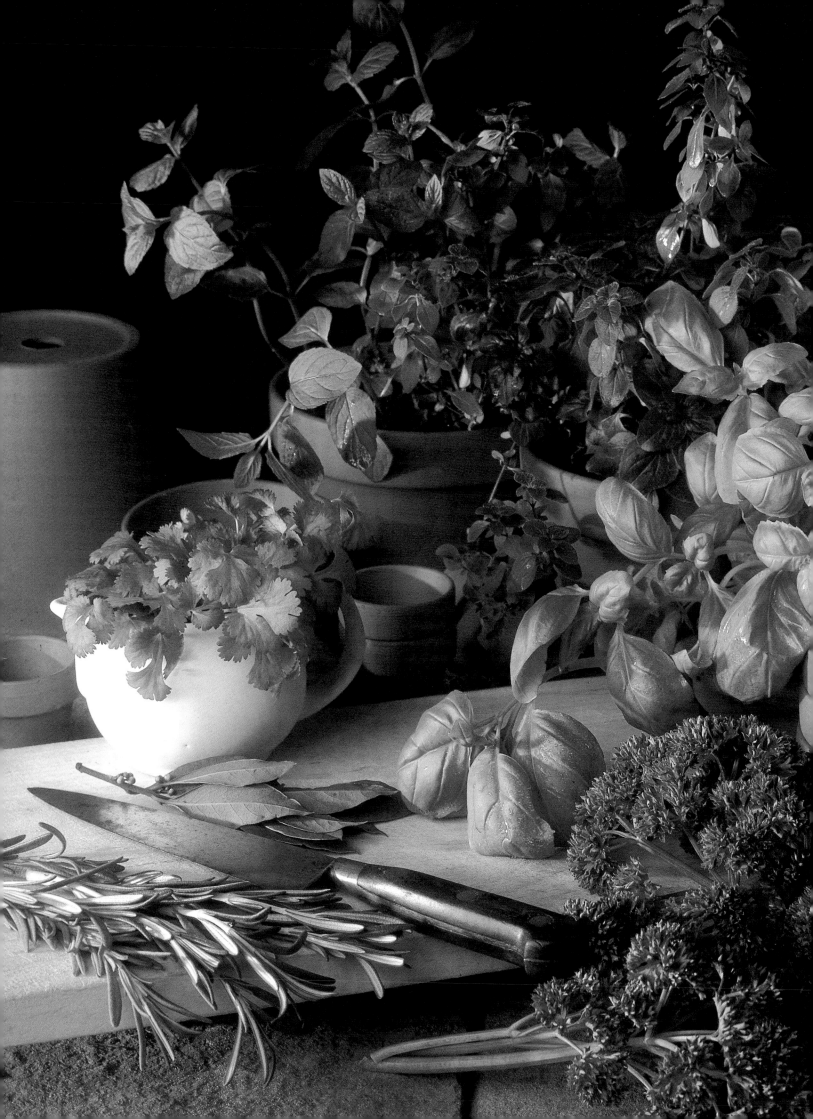

The Guide to
NATURAL THERAPIES

*Choosing and using natural methods
for physical and mental well-being*

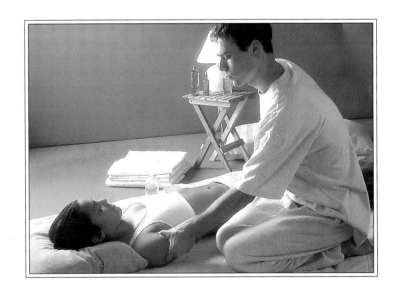

MARK EVANS B PHIL., FNIMH

SMITHMARK

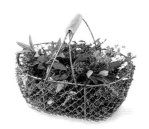

First published in 1996 by Smithmark Publishers Inc
a division of US Media Holdings Inc
16 East 32nd Street, New York, NY 10016

Produced by
Anness Publishing Limited
Hermes House
88-89 Blackfriars Road
London SE1 8HA

Publisher: Joanna Lorenz
Project Editor: Joanne Rippin
Designer: Nigel Partridge
Photographer: Don Last
Photographer's Assistant: Penny Hayler
Stylist: Susan Bull
Illustrations: Felicity Roma Bowers

Printed in Singapore by Star Standard Industries Pte Ltd

1 3 5 7 9 10 8 6 4 2

Additional text supplied by: John Hudson (Hypnotherapy), Andrew Oldroyd
(Moxibustion), Susan Franzen (Shiatsu), Karine Butchart (Makko Ho), Felicity Roma Bowers
(Meditation), Paul Harvey (Yoga), Anne Gains (Healthy Eating Plan), Clare Harris (Massage).

Additional photographs supplied by: Jacqui Hurst: p9. Michelle Garrett p8, 17, 21, 25, 27,
32, 33, 37. Lucy Mason p10, 11. Jean-Loup Charmet, Paris, p10. Mary Evans Picture Library p11,
48, 49, 60. Debbie Patterson p22. Tony Stone: Bruce Ayres p30, 52: Gary Brettnacher p38:
Timothy Shonnard p52. The Image Bank: Chris Close p51: Steve Satushek p55.

CONTENTS

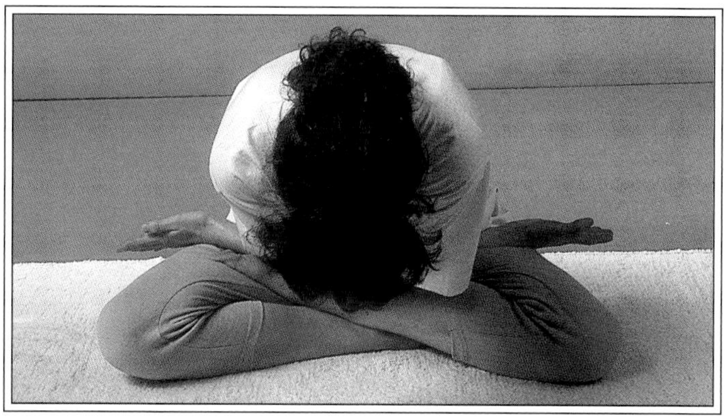

Chapter One

HEALTH FROM PLANTS 8

HERBAL MEDICINE 10

AROMATHERAPY 20

BACH FLOWER REMEDIES 26

HOMEOPATHY 27

Chapter Two

NATUROPATHY 28

DIET AND EXERCISE 30

HYDROTHERAPY 44

IRIDOLOGY 45

Chapter Three

STRESS MANAGEMENT 46

HYPNOTHERAPY 48

MEDITATION 54

PYSCHOTHERAPY 60

AUTOGENICS 62

HEALING 64

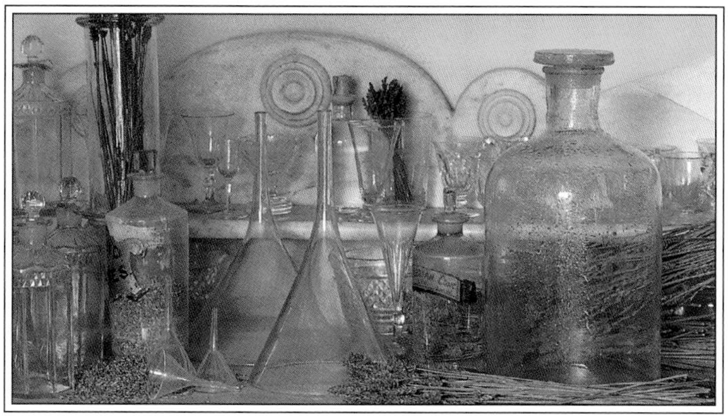

Chapter Four

BODYWORK 66

MASSAGE 68

ROLFING 79

REFLEXOLOGY 80

CHIROPRACTIC 84

CRANIO-SACRAL THERAPY 85

OSTEOPATHY 86

ALEXANDER TECHNIQUE 87

Chapter Five

EASTERN APPROACHES 88

SHIATSU 90

MAKKO HO 108

YOGA 114

MOXIBUSTION 124

CONTACTS AND ADDRESSES 127

INDEX 128

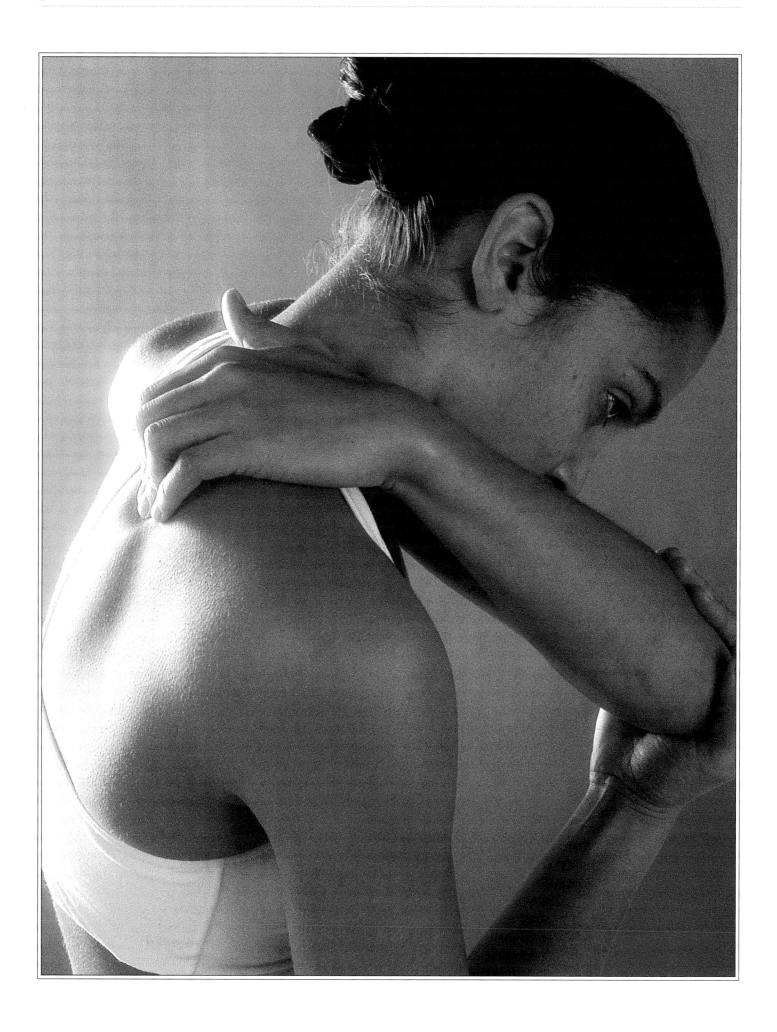

INTRODUCTION

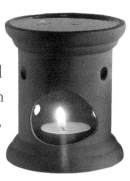

In a world of ever-increasing technology and machine-controlled medical interventions, people are beginning to feel the need for a human, individual touch; for a more natural approach to health that seeks to enhance life rather than dissect illness into more and more obscure diseases. Fortunately, there are a number of natural therapies which have just such a positive, holistic approach, and have also stood the test of

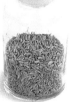

time, to emerge as the most rational way to sustain our health into the twenty-first century.

We have become accustomed to thinking of medicine as a crisis treatment for when we are sick, but one of the strengths of these therapies is their value in countering the effects of stress and helping to actually prevent illness. By reducing the impact of worries and stresses, many natural systems of treatment work to restore our vital energy and inner harmony.

Many Eastern cultures, such as those of China and India, have retained a strong tradition of therapies aimed at balancing energy, and in recent years these have gained increasing attention in the West. Our own traditional forms of treatment, such as herbalism and massage, have also undergone a resurgence in popularity, and lately there have been the beginnings of major research projects which confirm their value. Natural therapies not only have a long history, they have a bright future.

HEALTH FROM PLANTS

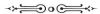

The most basic and the most pervasive source of medicines throughout the world ever since time began has been the plant kingdom. From our earliest origins we can trace the use of plants for health; even today most people rely on herbal medicines for most of their primary health care.

In ancient cultures, diet and medicine were inextricably linked – let your food be your medicine, and your medicine be your food – and the importance of diet to health is discussed in another section, but plants provide an additional healthy element to our food. Herbs not only enhance the flavour of what we eat, but often contain useful trace elements and also help with the digestion of many foods. Herbal teas are low-caffeine drinks that carry many health benefits too.

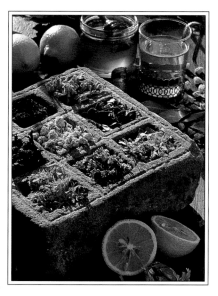

Professional herbal medicine may use plants with quite profound effects on our systems, while other therapies such as homoeopathy utilize the energetic qualities of plants, among other substances. In aromatherapy, the essential oils of plants are used to affect our emotional states, as well as for quite powerful anti-infective properties. As well as these therapies, requiring treatment from qualified practitioners, the plant world also offers many home remedies, and equally importantly plants can be used in many ways to maintain good health. This section shows some of these ways, and when to seek help.

ABOVE: A selection of herbs and dried flowers used in teas and tisanes.

OPPOSITE: A garden overflowing with plants used for centuries for their health-giving and medicinal qualities.

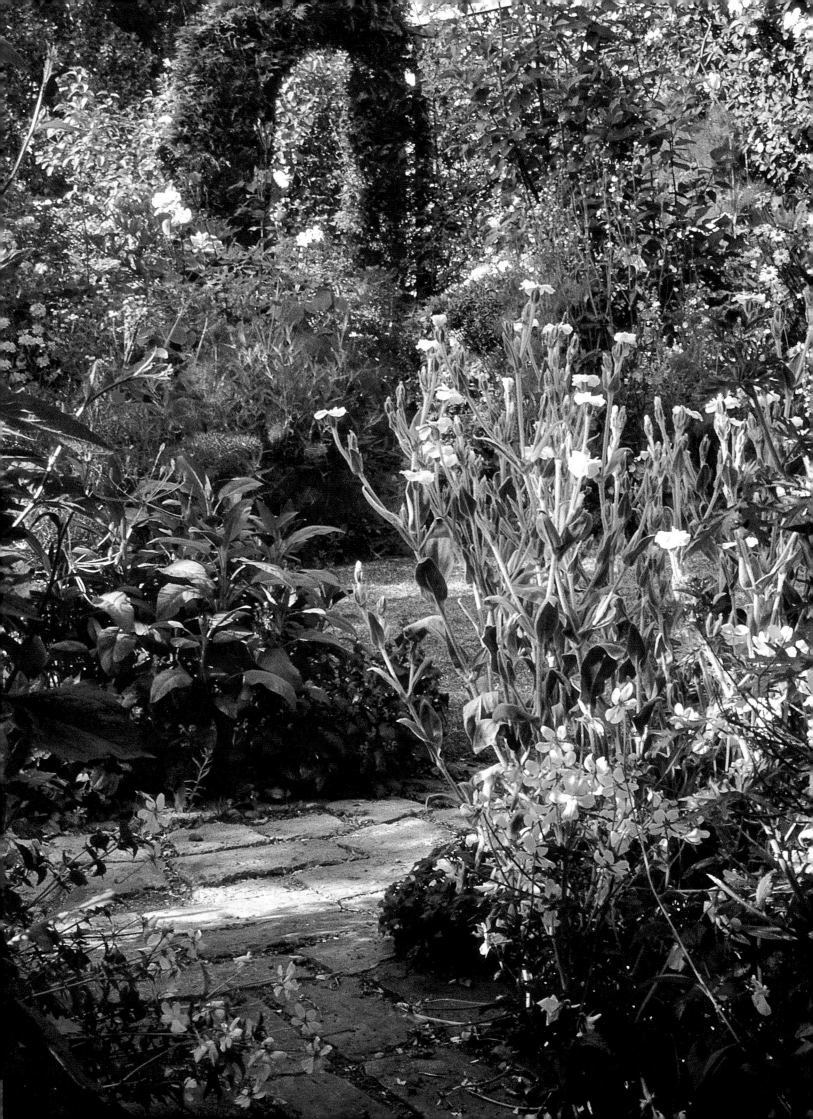

HERBAL MEDICINE

HISTORY AND ORIGINS

The history of herbal medicine is really the history of humankind, for every culture throughout time has relied upon herbs for its medicines. Some cultures – for instance, in India and China – have maintained a strong, unbroken tradition of herbalism for several centuries, while in Europe and North America its popularity has soared and plunged periodically as Western medicine achieved greater prominence. Today, however, interest in herbal medicine has increased once more, with an appreciation of its safer, holistic approach.

Probably the first system of herbal medicine, apart from the almost instinctive use of plants for healing that existed from the dawn of history and is still practised by remote tribes, was developed in India well over 4,000 years ago.

From India, the use of plants probably travelled with

BELOW: Although drying herbs alters their colour and flavour some, such as rosemary and thyme, keep many of their properties.

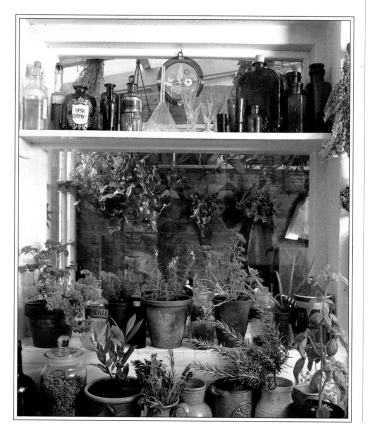

RIGHT: Ma-Kou (a Chinese goddess) carrying her medicinal herbs.

migrating people into China; traditional Chinese medicine has developed a strong philosophical viewpoint on health and disease, with treatments ranging from herbal medicines to acupuncture, moxibustion and massage techniques.

Knowledge also travelled westwards, into the Middle East, and one of the significant influences on present-day European herbalism was the ancient Egyptian tradition. Papyri dating back some 3,500 years indicate that the Egyptians used several hundred plants for food and medicine. These two uses were inextricably linked for centuries, as one Greek writer put it: "Let your food be your medicine, and your medicine be your food."

As the ancient Greeks expanded their empire, so their knowledge and use of herbs was spread throughout the realm, and other plants were added to their *materia medica*. When the Romans superseded the Greeks, their army doctors carried herbs and herbal medicine all over the known world. A large number of Mediterranean herbs were thus spread through Europe and into Britain. During these two great civilizations, several major works were written on natural history and medicine which were to be fundamental to medical thought for centuries.

After the decline of the Roman Empire, much of its literature went eastwards to Byzantium and the Arabic cultures. Traditional medicine here has retained a good deal of this ancient philosophy, and some of it came back to Europe with the Moorish invasions.

After the printing press was invented, all the old Greek

RIGHT: A traditional monastic layout is recreated in this twentieth-century garden, well stocked with a wide variety of herbs. Medieval monks kept physic gardens, growing herbs to make medicines for themselves and the local people, while the villagers would generally use simple plant treatments for all manner of ailments.

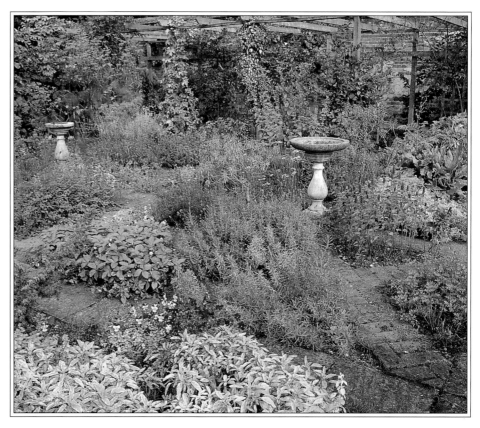

and Roman texts could be reproduced for a much wider readership. This coincided with the rapid expansion of towns and cities, and for the next three hundred years or so, knowledge and interest in herbs, in all areas of life, was greatly increased. By the sixteenth century, books about herbs were being published in the contemporary languages rather than Latin, and herbalism was an integral part of life. Books by authors such as Matthiolus, Turner, Gerard and Culpeper became bestsellers with practical advice on the uses of herbs; indeed Culpeper has never been out of print to this day, for over three hundred years.

Meanwhile, herbal medicines had been taken over by the settlers to America and used much as in Europe. It is possible to trace the spread of herbs along the eastern seaboard of the United States of America from early plantings by these settlers. Some of the more inquisitive migrants tried to learn from the Native Americans, since they were, before the importation of different diseases by the colonists, a healthy race.

The Native American system of health relied upon the use of herbs, simple yet nourishing food, fresh air and exercise. They also successfully used heat and water applications such as sweat lodges – teepees heated by a fire – with their physical and spiritual benefits.

The last ten to twenty years have seen another great resurgence in interest in natural medicine, and herbalism is both highly popular and increasingly respected as a safe and effective system of general medicine.

While today's professional practitioner of herbal medicine may see a wide range of people, often suffering from serious and chronic ill-health, the emphasis is always on the individual, looking at the whole picture of a person's health and not just any specific symptoms; this holistic approach is one good reason for its renewed popularity. Herbalism is also equally concerned with prevention or maintaining good health outside times of illness, and it is this aspect which attracts many people to use herbs in their daily lives.

LEFT: Native Americans used sweat lodges – teepees with a fire inside – as part of their natural medicine treatments.

HERBS IN FOOD

A number of widely used herbs have appreciable amounts of vitamins, minerals and trace elements, and can be thought of almost as nutritional supplements. Many others have excellent digestive qualities, helping the body cope with oily, fatty or gas-producing foods. For these reasons, as well as the extra pleasure given by their flavour, one of the earliest and best uses of herbs to help maintain health is in one's food.

LEAFY HERBS

BASIL, BAY, CORIANDER LEAVES, MARJORAM, MINT, OREGANO, PARSLEY, ROSEMARY, SAGE, SORREL, THYME.

These plants are essential ingredients in many culinary traditions, for their flavour and digestive properties. Most of these leafy herbs aid digestion, stimulating the production of enzymes that help break down fatty foods and aid absorption.

Mint sauce for example, traditionally used with lamb, helps to make this fatty meat easier to digest. Rosemary is often used with similar dishes for the same reason, stimulating the liver to work more effectively. Soups and stews are made much more tasty by the use of bay, marjoram or thyme; their aroma gets the digestive juices flowing before you have started the meal.

BASIL *(Ocimum basilicum)*

Most of these herbs contain important trace elements, and

BELOW: Sage, mint, rosemary and chives; herbs used in fresh and dried form for cooking and in salads.

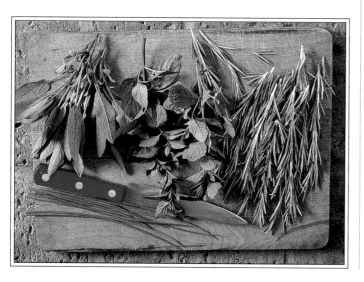

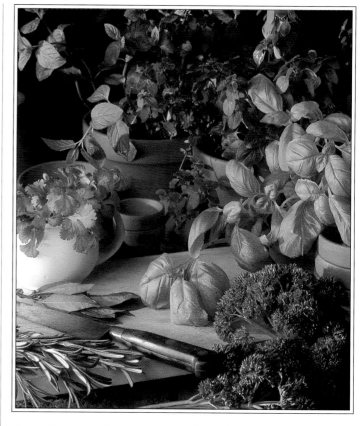

ABOVE: Leaves such as rosemary and parsley are essential in many culinary traditions for their flavour and as aids to digestion.

if the diet is restricted or lacking in nourishment then these nutrients can be very important in maintaining health. The herbs then become foods in themselves, and may be used in larger amounts such as in a sauce.

Parsley for instance is rich in iron and other minerals, while sorrel is a useful source of Vitamin C. Neither should be used all the time, but may add to the nutritional value of a meal. Like many other herbs, sage is a mild antiseptic and has a wide medicinal application in liver disease and respiratory tract infections. The oil is used in both the pharmaceutical and culinary industries.

CORIANDER *(Coriandrum sativum)*

The best way to benefit from herbs is to grow them yourself so that you always have a fresh supply. All the herbs mentioned above are easy to grow. You can even grow herbs inside on a sunny windowsill. Concentrate on the more common ones first and expand your collection as you go.

AROMATIC SEEDS

ANISEED, CARAWAY, CARDAMOM, CORIANDER, CUMIN, DILL, FENNEL, STAR ANISE.

These aromatic seeds are all to some extent carminative, that is they help almost immediately to reduce the build-up of excessive wind in the digestive tract, and to release any trapped gas. They have tradition-ally been used with foods that are notorious in creating wind. This carminative

ANISEED (Pimpinella anisum)

BELOW: To make the most of the beautiful fragrances and flavours of aromatic seeds, grind them in a pestle and mortar as required.

CUMIN *(Cuminum cyminum)*

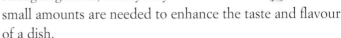

effect is contained within the essential oils in the seeds, and they have quite strong fragrances; usually only small amounts are needed to enhance the taste and flavour of a dish.

Caraway is a good example: used with foods such as cooked cabbage (a traditional association in Germany) or baked apples, it helps to prevent the bloating and discomfort that these can produce from trapped wind. Dill and fennel have been major ingredients in gripe water for babies for centuries, easing colicky pains. Coriander and cumin are important flavourings in curries and other Eastern dishes.

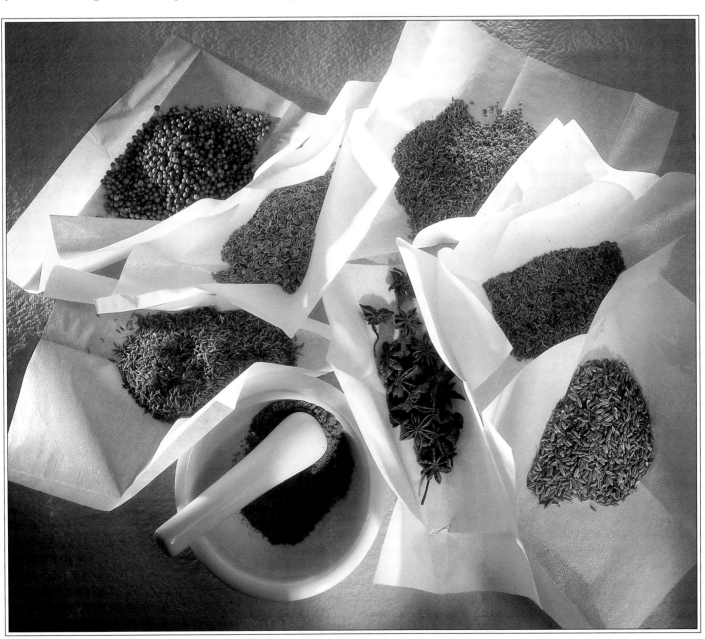

FRUITS AND BULBS

CHILLI PEPPERS, GARLIC, JUNIPER, PEPPERCORNS.

The general effects of these fruits is to speed up metabolism or to act as an antiseptic. Chilli peppers and peppercorns are both highly stimulating to the circulation; the effect of creating temporary heat in the stomach is to encourage gastric secretions, which in turn kill off potentially harmful bacteria in food. Traditionally this meant these herbs could be used in foods that might otherwise be toxic, the herbs providing protection as well as flavour.

RIGHT AND BELOW: The pungency of garlic and other fruits and bulbs such as chilli, juniper berries and peppercorns speeds up the metabolism and acts as an antiseptic.

RIGHT: Fresh green chilli.

The classic herb in this respect is garlic, which is not only warming, but helps lower cholesterol levels and fight infections. Juniper too is a powerful digestive antiseptic. Eating spicy, hot foods can make you perspire more, and this actually has a cooling effect which has long been appreciated by the inhabitants of hot countries.

Garlic and juniper have a traditional association with meats such as pheasant or hare, not just because their strong flavour calls for stronger-tasting herbs but because game can often be on the verge of going off. Any contamination is minimized by the antiseptic herbs.

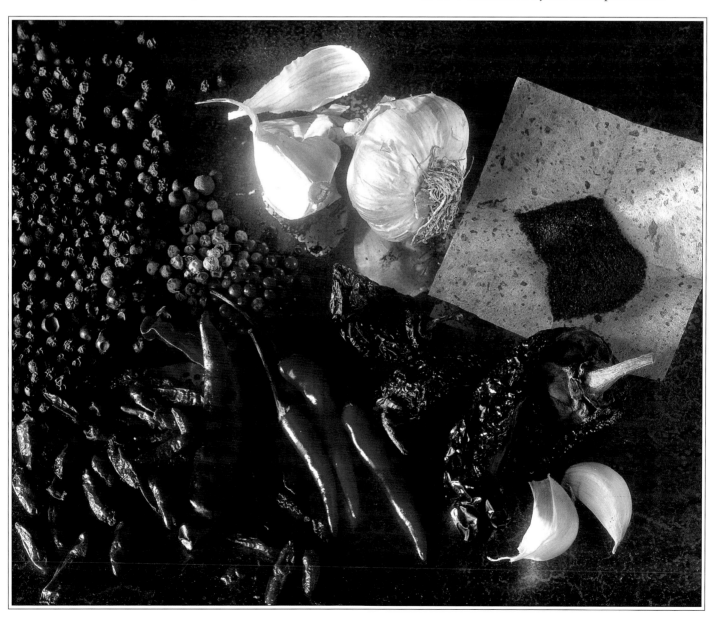

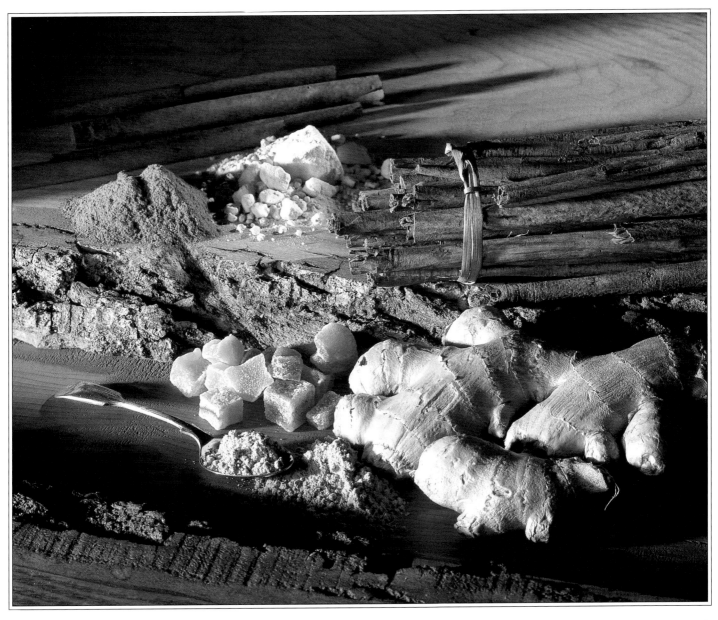

ROOTS AND BARK

CINNAMON, GINGER, HORSERADISH.

These are all circulatory stimulants, creating an inner warmth and vigour that can be very useful in colder climates. By speeding up the metabolism, blood moves around the body better and keeps our energy levels higher. In the digestive system, the transient heat that is created helps both with digestion and in reducing trapped wind. Generally, the increased circulation helps the immune system to work better, and these herbs can be used in foods over the cold months of the year to increase the body's natural resistance to colds. Horseradish has a pungent

GINGER (*Zingiber officinale*)

ABOVE: The warmth and spiciness of ginger in all its forms is used in many herbal remedies.

flavour that lends itself to savoury dishes, the classic combination being with roast beef. It is a stimulant and a weak diuretic. Ginger is much more versatile, and will go well with savoury rice dishes and apple pies for instance. Cinnamon is also often used in both savoury and sweet dishes, its own sweetness perhaps making it more useful for puddings. It has a less hot effect than the other two, gently warming the whole system.

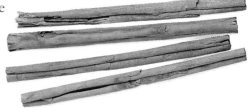

CINNAMON
(*Cinnamomum zeylanicum*)

HERB TEAS

One of the most widespread methods of using herbs to maintain good health and ward off illnesses is by drinking herb teas, or tisanes as they are known in France. For medicinal purposes, when treating an actual ailment, stronger preparations such as infusions or decoctions are prescribed, but in general it is possible to make a simple tisane at home.

Herb teas can be used as everyday hot drinks, to replace tea and coffee and hence reduce the caffeine intake in the diet. As each herb differs greatly in taste and flavour, it is very much an individual choice. A couple that have some of the taste qualities of ordinary tea are rooibosch and maté. The former has long been the daily drink for many people in South Africa, and is now grown in several countries; it makes a very enjoyable, low-caffeine tea. Similarly, maté is well-known in South American countries for its refreshing effect, with a smoky flavour reminiscent of Lapsang Souchong tea.

In general, it is sensible to vary herb teas, not only to enjoy a variety of flavours but to ensure that their medicinal properties are not overdone. Some can, however, be drunk over some considerable time, to maintain health and prevent ailments. In winter, especially in cooler climates, rose-hips might be a good choice. These contain considerable amounts of Vitamin C, which is an excellent way to sustain resistance to colds, flu and so on. Vitamin C can have something of a laxative effect, but the tannin content of rose-hips helps to balance this out. Many of the early naturopathic clinics in

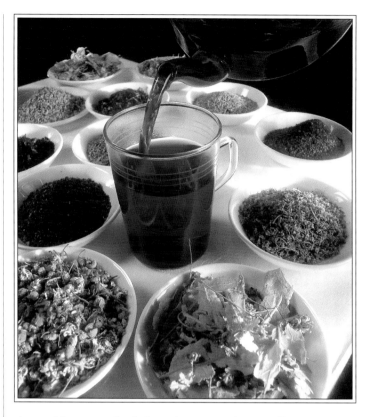

ABOVE: Most warm herbal teas have a comforting effect and are very easy to prepare.

Switzerland, such as that run by Dr Bircher-Benner, the creator of muesli, insisted that their clients drank a few cups of rose-hip tea daily. Tea bags are easily available in many countries and are very convenient to use, although quality varies.

A SIMPLE TISANE

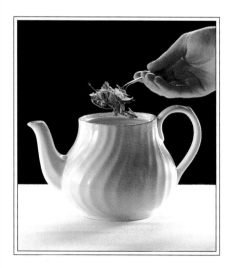

1 Warm a teapot and add one heaped teaspoonful of dried herb per person, or double for fresh herbs.

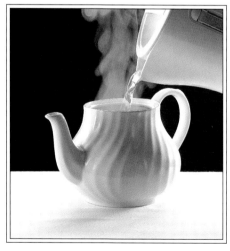

2 Pour on boiling water and allow to infuse for 2–3 minutes.

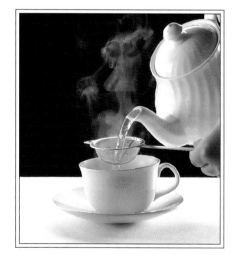

3 Strain and drink without milk or sugar (if you prefer a sweetener, use a little honey).

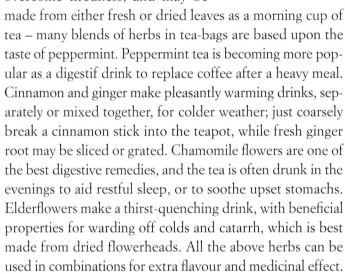

Mint (*Mentha x piperita*)

DANDELION TEA

Dandelions are a diuretic and can help to reduce water retention and bloated feelings. They can also help rheumatism. This tea acts as a mild laxative so should not be drunk in large quantities.

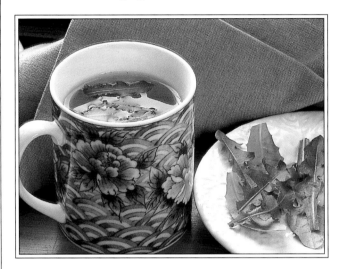

1 Remove any stems from the dandelion leaves. Tear them into strips and place in the bottom of a mug. Pour on enough boiling water to fill the mug and leave to stand for 5–10 minutes.

2 Strain, discard most of the dandelion leaves and drink. If you prefer a sweetener, add a small teaspoonful of honey.

A pleasant summer tea can be made from fresh lemon balm leaves: gather a few sprigs of the leaves, and make a tea, leaving it to stand for a few minutes. This herb reduces the impact of stress and anxiety on the system, especially where nervous indigestion is involved, and its balancing effects make it suitable for morning or evening drinking. The dried herb can be used too, but its flavour is inferior.

In hot weather, keep a jug of the tea in the refrigerator, perhaps with a slice or two of lemon for added flavour, and drink as you wish.

Peppermint and rosemary are both good pick-me-up teas, to prevent or overcome tiredness, and may be made from either fresh or dried leaves as a morning cup of tea – many blends of herbs in tea-bags are based upon the taste of peppermint. Peppermint tea is becoming more popular as a digestif drink to replace coffee after a heavy meal. Cinnamon and ginger make pleasantly warming drinks, separately or mixed together, for colder weather; just coarsely break a cinnamon stick into the teapot, while fresh ginger root may be sliced or grated. Chamomile flowers are one of the best digestive remedies, and the tea is often drunk in the evenings to aid restful sleep, or to soothe upset stomachs. Elderflowers make a thirst-quenching drink, with beneficial properties for warding off colds and catarrh, which is best made from dried flowerheads. All the above herbs can be used in combinations for extra flavour and medicinal effect.

Used regularly, herbal teas can make a significant contribution to a person's quality of health and wellbeing, not simply as replacements for stimulants such as tea or coffee, but for their general health-giving properties and specific medicinal benefits.

HERB TEA CHART

Herb	Property	Benefit
Chamomile	Relaxant, digestive, anti-inflammatory	Settles digestion, aids restful sleep
Cinnamon	Carminative, warming, diaphoretic	Improves digestion and good when cold/chilled
Elderflower	Expectorant, diaphoretic	Clears catarrh, reduces fevers by sweating
Lemon Balm	Relaxant, digestive, anti-depressant	Relieves nervous dyspepsia, good tonic
Lime Blossom	Relaxant, analgesic	Eases tension headaches or aching colds and flu
Peppermint	Antispasmodic and digestive	Reduces flatulence, is good for head colds too
Rosehip	Contains Vitamin C	Helps build resistance to colds and flu

HERB SUPPLEMENTS

All in all, therefore, herbs can play an essential role in maintaining one's health and vitality on a daily basis. They provide much more than extra flavouring to food, enjoyable though this may be, and their continued and universal popularity demonstrates how much people rely on them to keep well. Many herbs can be used as effective, powerful yet safe remedies for all kinds of ailments.

Herbs in other forms can also be used to maintain good health. Many people's experience of herbal medicines is in the form of tablets or capsules obtained from health stores or other outlets. Some of these extracts are more valuable in preventing ill-health than as medications; if you are actually ill, it may be better to consult a herbal practitioner since the principle of herbalism is based on individual treatment.

GARLIC

One of the most effective herbal remedies is garlic, which can help tremendously in building up resistance to respiratory infections, warding off colds, flu and so on. Garlic needs to be taken daily during the late autumn, winter and early spring months to sustain this resistance. Undoubtedly it is most effective when a fresh bulb is used, ideally raw, but as you can lose most of your friends if taking garlic this way every day, it may be more suitable to take one of the commercial garlic capsules that are

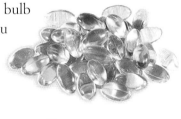

GARLIC TABLETS

easily found. These are less powerful, but should impart less odour to the breath – the reason for garlic's actions in resisting respiratory infections is that the (smelly) essential oil which gives it a powerful antiseptic property is 99 per cent excreted via the lungs.

ECHINACEA

Another herb with very useful properties is *Echinacea* (sometimes called purple coneflower). This stimulates the immune system, boosting general resistance to infection and illness. If vitality has been lowered, or if you simply wish to strengthen the immune response, *Echinacea* is available in either a liquid form or as tablets (sometimes it can be found combined with garlic), and a course may be taken for three or four weeks to raise immunity.

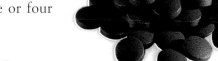

GINSENG TABLETS

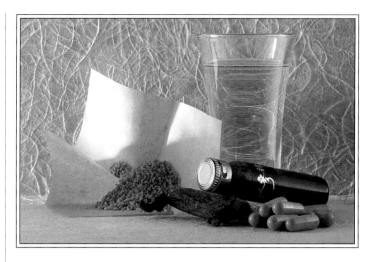

ABOVE: Ginseng, renowned in China as a powerful natural remedy for hundreds of years, is now used more and more in the West.

GINSENG

Chronic stress is one major source of impaired immunity, and it may well be useful before or during a time of increased stress, or indeed before the winter arrives in colder climates, to take a three-week course of herbs to improve your ability to cope with physical, emotional and mental stresses. The classic herbs for this are the various ginsengs. These are most suitable for waning energy and are to be used with caution (if at all) where people respond to stress with increased anxiety or tension and raised blood pressure. Korean, or Asiatic ginseng (*Panax schinseng*), gives the most uplift, while American ginseng (*P. quinquefolium*) has a more relaxing effect. Siberian ginseng (*Eleutherococcus senticosus*) is a completely different plant, with similar effects to Korean ginseng in enhancing stamina. These are all available as tablets, and the two *Panax* species can often be found as the actual dried root, which may be chewed in small pieces or made into a tea.

EVENING PRIMROSE

A plant that has become very popular in recent years is the evening primrose; the oil extracted from the seeds is a potent source of essential fatty acids, particularly a substance called gamma-linoleic acid. Some people do not produce enough of this compound, which in turn can lead to a shortage of more complex compounds that have beneficial effects in a number of ailments, such as arthritis, eczema and even multiple sclerosis. Evening primrose oil, however, is perhaps best known and most widely used for its use in helping ease premenstrual problems or the symptoms of the menopause. Obviously, the full treatment of hormonal disorders requires professional attention, but there may be a case for taking evening primrose oil capsules daily (500–1500mg) as a preventive treatment in the early stages of the menopause.

FEVERFEW

Another good self-help herb to use in order to help prevent the occurrence, or recurrence, of ailment symptoms is feverfew. This is another plant which has gained in popularity, this time for its usefulness in warding off migraines. It is not to be thought of as a remedy to take when you have a

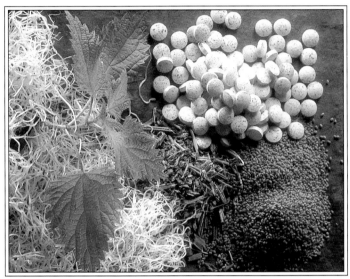

migraine – the reasons for which can often be a detective story and need individual treatment – but as a preventive measure. The herb is now widely available in tablet form, daily dosage about 125mg, and as the fresh leaves taste very bitter and can occasionally cause mouth ulcers, the tablets are a convenient way to use feverfew.

ALFALFA AND KELP

Some herbs are sufficiently rich in nutrients to be thought of as food supplements, although it may be more appropriate to use them in different ways. Sprouted alfalfa, for instance, contains high amounts of several vitamins and minerals; this is best taken as part of the diet, eaten in salads where it gives a crunchy bite to the dish. Nettles are very rich in iron, together with some Vitamin C, and can make an energy-giving tea for people who are bordering on being anaemic. Kelp contains several minerals, notably iodine which acts as a tonic for the thyroid gland, and can aid those who have a sluggish metabolism; this herb should *not* be used by anyone taking thyroxine for an under-active thyroid gland – if in doubt, seek professional advice. Many seaweeds are used in cooking, especially in Japanese cuisine, and this is one way to take them; kelp is also easily found in tablet form, and this is a useful way to take a daily course for, say, four weeks to boost the system.

ABOVE: Clockwise from top left: alfalfa sprouts, nettles, kelp tablets, alfalfa seeds and dried kelp.

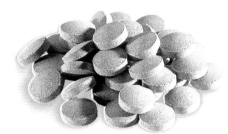

KELP TABLETS

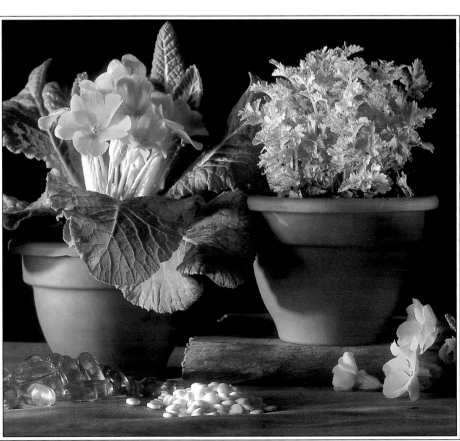

RIGHT: Evening primrose is widely used to alleviate the side-effects of menstruation.

AROMATHERAPY

HISTORY

One of the most primitive forms of medicine involved burning aromatic plants in order to "smoke" illness out of a patient. This process was frequently interlinked with various rituals and religious practices, and sometimes plants with mind-altering properties were burnt too, to create a mystical, other-worldly experience as part of the healing ritual. The use of incense in the ceremonies of diverse religions through the centuries has perpetuated this aspect; many of the gums and resins that are used in incense have powerful therapeutic properties – for example, as respiratory antiseptics – as well as inducing a meditative, reflective state of mind in the worshippers.

Aromatic plants and extracts have been highly regarded by all the greater ancient civilizations, stretching through the Middle East from Babylonia and Persia to India and China. The oldest medical texts from these countries, dating back at least 3,000 years, list many aromatic plants and their uses. Some of the most detailed descriptions are to be found in ancient Egyptian writings; fragrant plants were employed in all aspects of life, from perfume and cosmetics to medicine and in the rituals for embalming the dead. Some of the ointment jars excavated from Tutankhamen's tomb contained

BELOW: Aromatherapy oils are now widely available and can be mixed with pure vegetable oils for use in massage.

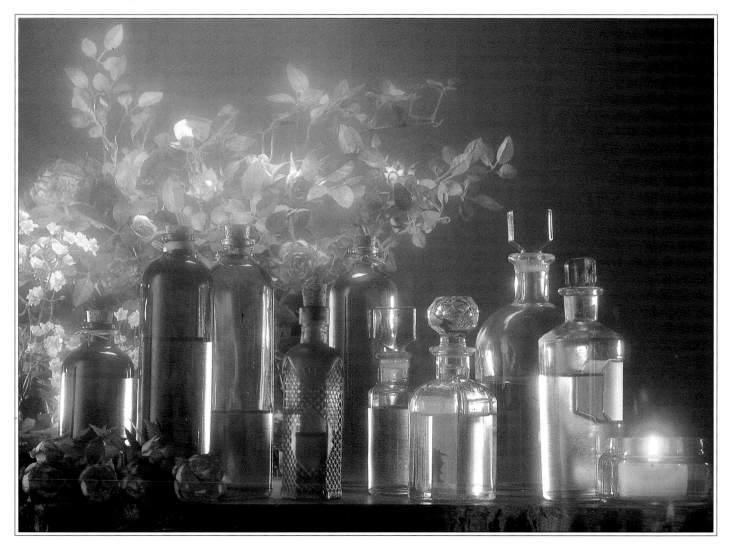

preservative resins such as frankincense which still had an odour after some 3,200 years.

The Egyptians were very aware of the value of fragrance in enhancing mood, and developed a reputation as masters of perfumery; Cleopatra may have owed something of her fabled attractiveness to Julius Caesar and Mark Antony from her use of vast amounts of rose petals to scent her living quarters. Interestingly, however, the Egyptians do not appear to have discovered the process of distilling the essential oils from plants, relying instead on infused oils and ointments. These were later widely used by the Greeks and Romans, both as medicine and as part of the daily ritual of public bathing, which the Romans in particular so enjoyed.

Many Greek physicians were employed by the Roman armies, and they carried the knowledge of aromatic, and other, plants across many countries. Galen, who rose to be the personal physician to the Emperor Marcus Aurelius, invented the original cold cream and was a great writer on all matters concerning health and medicines. His and other works formed the basis of medicine for many centuries, and with the decline of the Roman Empire much of this knowledge went eastwards into Byzantium. It was the Arabic countries that made the next great leap forwards in aromatherapy. By the ninth century, Baghdad was thriving partly due to being the centre of the rose industry, exporting rose water as far as India. The principle of distillation was first applied to roses and is generally credited to Abu Ali Ibn Sina, better known as Avicenna (980–1037), a philosopher and physician from Uzbekistan. Steam distillation enabled the pure essential oil to be extracted from many plants.

In the West, aromatic infused oils had continued to be used, and during the period of the Crusades, essential oils, or "perfumes of Arabia" as they were known, spread extensively throughout Europe. As the gums and resins of Asia were not easily available, native Mediterranean plants such as rosemary and lavender were used for making essential oils too. The French were particularly enthusiastic in adopting these oils, laying the foundations for today's perfumery industry as well as therapeutic uses.

Burning antiseptic herbs such as thyme and rosemary, to fumigate the air and ward off disease, was carried out in several French hospitals until well into the twentieth century. Indeed, it was a Frenchman, René Gattefosse, a chemist working in the perfumery industry, who coined the term aromatherapy some 50 years ago. He burned his hand badly in an accident in his laboratory. He used essential oil of lavender to cool the tissue and found it healed the burned flesh remarkably quickly, with no infection or scar. During both

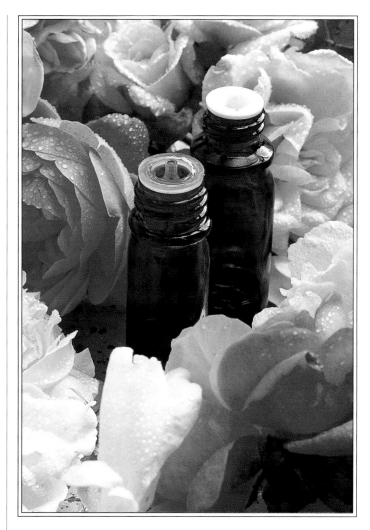

Above: Essential oils are highly concentrated; it can take 5,000 roses to produce just one teaspoonful of oil.

World Wars, essential oils were used to treat wounds and infections, and one of the pioneers of this work was Dr Jean Valnet, who published his findings in the late 1960s. Respected medical establishments in France are now looking at the medicinal aspects of essential oils.

It should not be forgotten, however, that the power of aromatic plants extends beyond antiseptic or anti-inflammatory properties. It is well established that scent can evoke memories, change people's moods and make them feel good. Aromatherapy has developed in the UK, the US and many other countries in the last 20 years into a holistic system that tries to heal and balance the whole person. The oils are often incorporated into massage, or used in baths, or simply evaporated into the air in a burner to improve physical and emotional well-being. These methods would all be familiar to the ancients, and show a continuing tradition of usage of aroma in therapy. There are also more aromatherapy practitioners than ever before offering complete treatments.

OILS AND PREVENTION

Many of the beauty and cosmetic products now on the market contain essential oils, their popularity stemming both from their wonderful fragrance and the widespread interest in using as many natural ingredients as possible. Aromatic essential oils can also be used in a number of ways to maintain good health and prevent ailments; it should always be remembered, however, that self-help is not a substitute for seeking professional treatment for an illness or condition. Furthermore, the pure essential oils themselves are highly concentrated and should be treated with respect. For instance, it may have taken 5,000 roses to produce a teaspoonful of essential oil of rose!

A useful guideline when using essential oils at home – for instance, in the bath – is the 1–2 rule. Use only one or two oils together at any time; use one or two drops in the bath; and do not use any particular oil on a daily basis for more than one or at most two weeks.

Some essential oils have a stimulating effect on the uterine muscles and should therefore not be used if you are pregnant, or suspect you might be. The possibly problematic oils to be avoided during your pregnancy include basil, clary sage, fennel, hyssop, juniper, pennyroyal, peppermint,

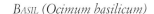

BASIL (Ocimum basilicum)

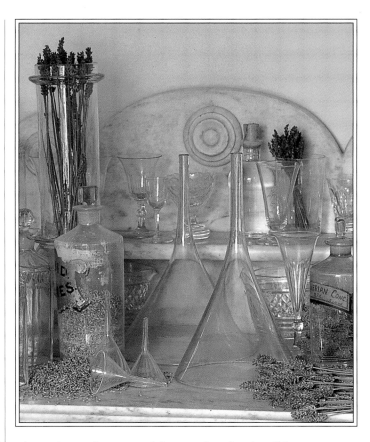

ABOVE: *Lavender is one of the most loved and well-known essential oils and has been distilled for centuries.*

sage and thyme. Equally, if you ever get any skin irritation or allergic reaction to any oil, then you should of course stop using it. Many of these herbs are used in cooking and are quite safe for pregnant women in this form.

ESSENTIAL THERAPIES

AROMATHERAPY OIL	PROPERTIES AND BENEFITS
Lavender	Antiseptic, anti-depressant, healing; relieves stress and insomnia, soothes insect bites.
Rose	Anti-depressant, aphrodisiac, tonic; helpful for menstrual disorders; aids sleep.
Bergamot	Antiseptic, astringent, stimulative; helps to combat oily skin but can sensitize it to UV light.
Sandalwood	Healing, antiseptic; can relieve fluid retention, cystitis and insomnia.
Patchouli	Healing, soothing; helps combat dandruff and dry skin patches.
Ylang Ylang	Antiseptic, aphrodisiac, tonic.
Myrrh	Healing, antiseptic, calming; eases viral and fungal infections such as thrush (if added to a bath).
Juniper	Diuretic, antiseptic, cleansing, calming; avoid in first five months of pregnancy, not to be used by those with kidney disease.
Neroli	Calming; soothes nerves and upset stomachs; a good remedy for dry skin.
Chamomile, Roman	The most soothing oil; relieves anxiety, stress, allergies, and Pre-menstrual syndrome (PMS).
Basil	Reviving, decongestive.
Rosemary	Antiseptic, stimulating, balancing, diuretic, uplifting; not to be used in the first five months of pregnancy, or by those with high blood pressure.
Frankincense	Decongestive, relaxing; aids sleep.

OILS IN THE AIR

A widely used method of employing essential oils in the home is to fragrance the rooms by means of a vaporizer, or oil burner. Vaporizers are widely available, and range from the simple utilitarian version to the highly decorative, hand-crafted piece. Although they come in many forms, they all work on the same principle. The reservoir, or receptacle, is filled with water, to which are added drops of essential oil. The reservoir is then heated, causing the water to evaporate and the warm oil to release its perfume.

CHOOSING AND USING A VAPORIZER

When choosing a vaporizer there are two important points to consider. First, there should be a suitable distance between the source of the heat and the reservoir for oil and water. This will reduce the risk of completely evaporating the water and therefore burning the oil. Second, the vaporizer should be easy to clean, ready for use with a different oil.

The simplest type of vaporizer makes use of a candle as the heat source; a more efficient, but more expensive, type is the electric vaporizer. Under certain circumstances these are preferable to the type heated by a candle – for example in the reception area of an office, in a hospital ward, or at home, when you want to disperse oils for a long period of time without the necessity of frequent supervision. Some electric vaporizers have a silent fan that disperses the evaporating oils; others employ a heated ceramic dish. Either would be suitable for a child's bedroom, or a room occupied by someone who is bedridden.

Whenever you use a vaporizer of any kind, do make certain that you place the burner in a safe position, out of the reach of children and pets.

The number of drops of oil used in a burner depends on the size of the room: two to three drops for a small room, and as many as six to ten for a larger one. It is better to use fewer drops and refresh the burner more frequently, rather than use too many and saturate a room with scent. Remember too that your sensitivity to the scent will decrease, but this does not mean that the

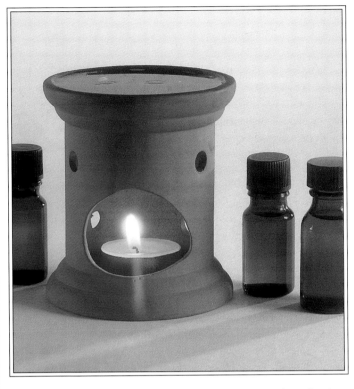

ABOVE: A terracotta vaporizer makes a lovely, warm, friendly glow as it burns and is as much a pleasure to look at as to smell.

aroma is not still present and probably still quite strong.

If you do not have a vaporizer, or you feel the need for an instant aromatherapy treatment, try applying just a few drops of oil to a handkerchief or paper towel and gently inhaling the perfume. Placing the handkerchief on your pillow at night should ease breathing if you have a blocked nose; some oils will help promote a good night's sleep. It is not wise to take essential oils as a medicine except on the advice of a practitioner, but some people do use essential oils in tea, adding two or three drops of a suitable oil to a pot of black tea for digestive problems, urinary problems or stress.

These are just some of the ways in which aromatherapy can be used as a preventive healthcare system in the home. In general, start with just a few oils, find out about their properties and uses, and go from there. One of the best things about aromatherapy is the pleasure to be derived from the aromas; keeping healthy can be enjoyable and fun.

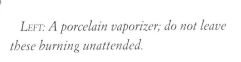

LEFT: A porcelain vaporizer; do not leave these burning unattended.

OIL IN WATER

One of the most pleasant ways of using aromatic oils is to put one or two drops into a bath just before you get in; they form a thin film over the surface of the water, which coats and penetrates the skin while you lie in the heady aroma. If you have very dry skin, try adding a couple of drops of your chosen essential oil to a teaspoonful of pure vegetable oil, such as sweet almond, and pour this into the bath.

To help ward off the effects of the cold in winter, try using oils that have a warming effect on the circulation, such as black pepper, ginger, marjoram or rosemary. These are especially good in the morning, to stimulate the whole system. Respiratory infections can be another problem of colder months, and using essential oils through the winter months can help to build resistance to colds, coughs and so on. Oils to consider here are benzoin, eucalyptus, frankincense, lavender, pine, tea-tree and thyme, as well as the circulatory stimulants mentioned above.

After the winter, many people can feel rather sluggish and perhaps be overweight. This can be a good time to use refreshing essential oils that also help to aid digestion. Among others, choose from fennel, geranium, grapefruit, lemon, mandarin and orange – most of these are citrus oils, which have an uplifting, stimulating quality.

On the emotional level, several essences have quite remarkable effects in helping to keep our moods in balance. The best anti-depressant oil is undoubtedly bergamot, and

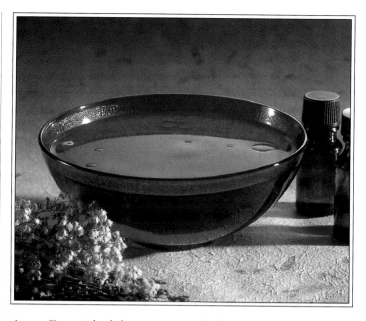

ABOVE: Essential oils have an ancient link with water and have been used since classical times as part of a bathing ritual.

this can be used to ward off low vitality at times of stress and depression. A note of caution though – bergamot increases sensitivity to the sun, so do not overuse before exposure to bright sunlight.

Other mood-elevators are neroli (or orange blossom), jasmine, melissa and rose. All of these particular oils are very expensive to produce, and this in itself gives a feeling of luxurious pampering when using them.

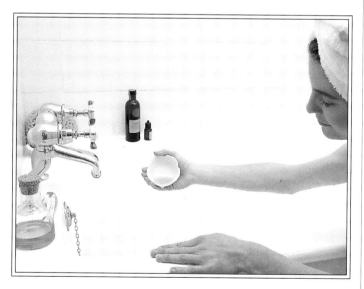

ABOVE: Add some pure vegetable oil and one to two drops of essential oil for a relaxing, steaming bath.

RIGHT: For a steam inhalation place ten drops of oil and a cup of hot water in a bowl. Inhale deeply through your nose.

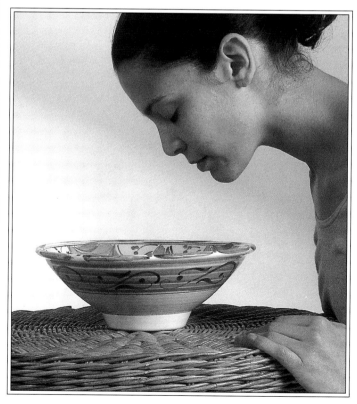

OILS IN MASSAGE

For direct use on the skin, essential oils must be diluted. Use a good, pure vegetable oil as the base, such as coconut, apricot kernel, jojoba (actually a liquid wax) or sweet almond. If your skin tends to be very dry, add about ten per cent of avocado or wheatgerm oil to the blend – avoid the latter if you are allergic to wheat. The essential oils are added at one or two per cent; assuming 20 drops to 1ml, this means using one or two drops per 5ml (1 tsp) of base oil.

All the above suggestions for bath oils apply equally to aromatherapy massage. Another area of use is in skincare itself. Some essential oils have a balancing, healing effect on the skin; frankincense, lavender, neroli, rose and sandalwood in particular can all be massaged into the skin regularly. It may be easier to mix them, at the same dilution, into your favourite skin cream; make up small amounts at a time, and vary them after a while.

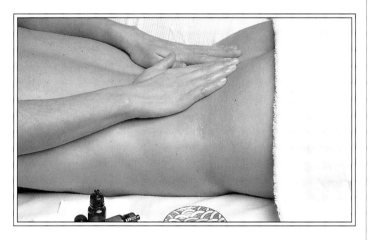

SPORTS BLENDS

The oils listed below are grouped according to their usefulness before and after sporting activities.

BEFORE
❦ For stimulation: juniper, eucalyptus and rosemary.
❦ For supple, toned muscles: black pepper, ginger, rosemary, lavender, cypress, juniper, peppermint, grapefruit, orange.
❦ To aid a good strong respiratory system for aerobics: eucalyptus, peppermint, rosemary, geranium.
❦ To aid mental preparation before a competition: a blend of rosemary, lemon, lavender, chamomile.
❦ To promote good circulation: rose and palmarosa.

AFTER
❦ To soothe and prevent aching muscles: eucalyptus, ginger and peppermint.
❦ To eliminate stress following a competition: lemon, nutmeg, clary sage, orange.

LEFT: Massaging with essential oils is a good way to appreciate their benefits.

BELOW: Remember to bring the oil to room temperature before you use it, to help release its precious aroma.

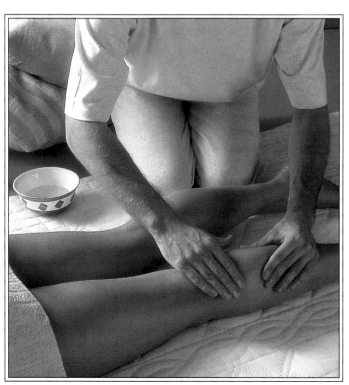

DILUTING OIL FOR MASSAGE

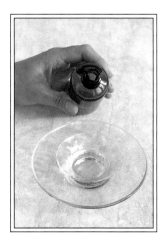
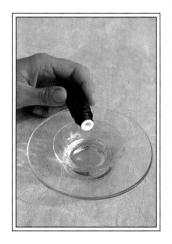

1 Pour the equivalent of two teaspoonsfuls of pure vegetable oil into a bowl.

2 Very carefully add one or two drops of essential oil and mix together.

BACH FLOWER REMEDIES

The Bach flower remedies are named after their originator, a Dr Edward Bach. He was a medical doctor, immunologist and bacteriologist who developed a successful practice in Harley Street, London, at the beginning of the twentieth century. After several years of practice, he became convinced that much of the medicine of his day was counter-productive, depressing rather than enhancing our natural self-healing energies. For some time he was interested in homeopathy, but eventually felt that remedies should only come from nature – plants, sunlight and pure water. He gave up his lucrative practice, moved to Wales and spent the rest of his life developing a range of gentle plant-based remedies.

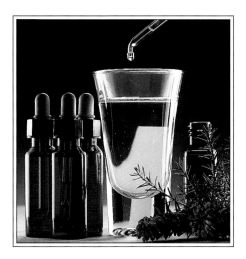

ABOVE: The flowers for the remedies are distilled in pure spring water.

Dr Bach seems to have been something of a sensitive or medium, because after he had a severe illness, he found that he had an ability to assess the healing properties of various plants intuitively. Over the years he had come to the conclusion that behind all illness was an inner imbalance, an emotional or psychological state that affected the individual's health. He also felt that the vital properties of a plant were transmitted into the dew that would form in the early morning, and that this essence could be captured by floating the plant on pure spring water and leaving it for a while in the sunlight. These preparations are then preserved with a little brandy, creating in effect a diluted tincture, although not as extremely diluted as homeopathic remedies.

The flower remedies are prescribed therefore to treat negative emotional moods or states of mind, whatever the physical complaint. Their effects are thus rather difficult to evaluate – it is easier to note the disappearance of physical symptoms than a change in emotional make-up – but although sometimes subtle, the remedies can have profound effects on people's vitality and health.

Remedies may be prescribed singly or in combinations, but generally the fewer taken at one time the better. It therefore requires honesty and sensitivity when deciding what negative emotional aspect is dominant at that point. Self-prescribing is certainly possible, and Bach himself intended these remedies to be simple enough, and safe enough, for people to use on themselves. The remedies are sold in small bottles with dropper inserts, and from these stock remedies one takes four drops a dose. These may either be placed straight on to the tongue, or diluted further with a little spring water and then sipped frequently. The dose may be repeated four times a day. The high level of dilution means that the Bach remedies are usually safe for children.

Interestingly, Rescue Remedy, a compound of five of his original remedies, has become very popular as one of the finest treatments for shock, even with people who know nothing about the other remedies. Although research has failed to come up with an explanation for the effectiveness of Bach remedies, it is accepted that there is a physiological basis for its benefits, and its popularity is growing.

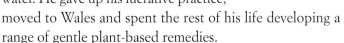

BELOW: An important part of developing Bach flower remedies is the application of sunlight and water to the plants.

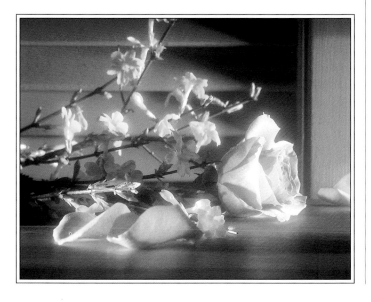

HOMEOPATHY

Homeopathy dates back to the end of the eighteenth century, although it has much earlier antecedents. A German doctor, Samuel Hahnemann, gave up his medical practice in the 1780s in protest at the violent measures then practised, such as bloodletting and strong purging. He felt that such treatments often made patients weaker than their original illness, and for a time he turned to making a living as a translator of medical works. While working on a herbal by a Scottish writer called Cullen, he came across the assertion that cinchona bark (from which quinine was later derived) was a helpful treatment for malaria because it was a good astringent.

Since there were plenty of better astringents available, Hahnemann decided to test cinchona bark on himself to see its effects. After a few days, he started to get all the symptoms of malaria, although he did not have the disease. This led Hahnemann to the concept that symptoms were not a sign of disease but an indication of the body's attempts to fight illness; the cinchona strengthened this response. To test

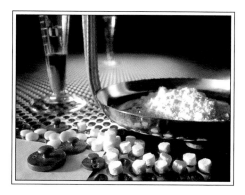

ABOVE: The distinctive little white homeopathic pills prescribed to stimulate the body's immune responses.

this theory further, he tried out many more medicines on himself, friends and others, and eventually came to the principle of *similia similibus curantur* – "like will cure like"; that is, a remedy which induces certain reactions in a healthy person will be a valuable remedy for treating an illness in which these same symptoms are seen.

Hahnemann also found that symptoms often seemed to get worse initially when people were given a remedy. In order to overcome this, he diluted his remedies in a special way until they became almost undetectable, and yet the therapeutic effect seemed to get stronger. He reasoned that the healing effects must be carried out on a subtle, energetic level. He termed his system homoeopathy, literally meaning "like disease".

HOMEOPATHIC PRINCIPLES

❧ Homeopathic remedies act by stimulating our immune responses into greater action, to bring about a cure.

❧ The remedy itself does not bring about a cure, this comes from within us.

❧ The correct remedy for someone is the one that when given to a healthy person produces the same symptoms as the disease is producing in the ill person.

❧ To reduce or avoid aggravations of the symptoms, the remedy should be given in very small dosages.

❧ Dilution of the remedy, accompanied by a vigorous shaking, acts in such a way as to potentize its effects; the greater the dilution, the quicker and more effective the remedy.

Remedies are often diluted using the centessimal scale, that is one part of the original substance is diluted and succussed with 99 parts of a liquid, usually alcohol or water. This would make a 1c potency. One part of this is then diluted with 99 parts of liquid for a 2c potency, and so on.

Homeopathy has been widely used in some countries for a long time; in the last 20 years, its popularity has increased across the world and it has become much more accepted.

BELOW: Marigolds are an important ingredient in homeopathy.

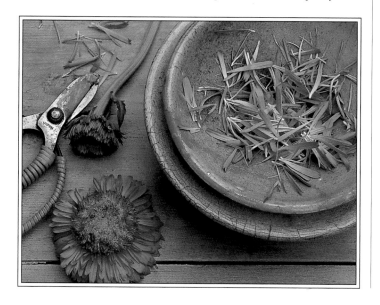

NATUROPATHY

This section is intended to cover those areas of self-help and professional therapies that do not fit into the other categories of this book. More than that, however, they comprise those approaches that focus on our natural healing abilities and try simply to enhance them. Iridology has been included here since it aims to diagnose imbalances by "reading" our own natural body signs, and treatment is often along naturopathic lines.

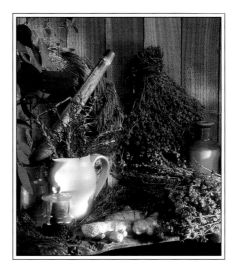

Naturopathy is itself a professional therapy, including diet, exercise, supplements and hydrotherapy within its field. Some traditions of naturopathic training also link with some of the hands-on professions such as osteopathy or chiropractic, and the practitioners of these latter disciplines may advocate other measures to help to restore full health. Hydrotherapy, or "water cure", has a strong tradition in Northern Europe, and is still carried out at centres in Germany, Austria, Switzerland and France. Increasingly it is also becoming more widespread in the US.

Both diet and exercise are vital elements in achieving and maintaining optimal health, and most of us can make adjustments in these areas. Some ideas for improvement are presented here; a key factor is to include exercises and dietary changes that you will enjoy, as a part of really appreciating life.

Above: A selection of natural herbs and plants.

Opposite: A balanced diet gives us a secure foundation for good health and vitality.

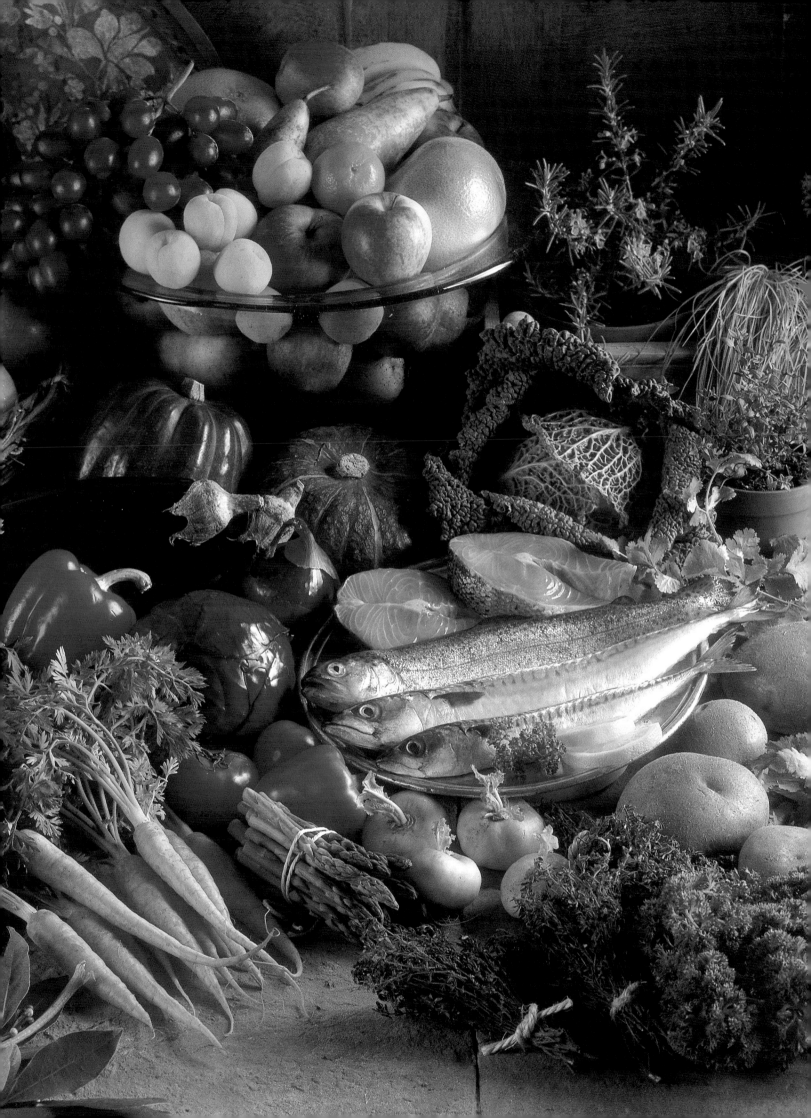

DIET AND EXERCISE

Probably the two most obvious and successful ways in which we can affect our health are through nutrition and exercise. Most of the natural therapies will include an assessment of and advice about these areas; indeed naturopathy focuses largely on them as a means of treating illness. A healthy diet and adequate exercise are essential for health, and although many books and magazines are devoted to encouraging us to work on these factors, they provide so much advice and differing theories and methods that it seems difficult to fulfil these aims.

A healthy diet involves eating foods that provide all the nourishment that our bodies need for growth, tissue repair, energy to carry out vital internal processes and to stay fit and active. In the last hundred years or so, the changes in eating habits in many countries have meant that large numbers of people have become overfed. Ironically, at the same time these dietary changes have left a lot of us undernourished, lacking in vitamins, minerals and trace elements that would help us to be in the peak of health.

Eating for health does not have to mean switching to a fussy, complicated diet, or adopting every new fad that comes

BELOW: Most people find it more stimulating to exercise in a group and there are many different classes to choose from.

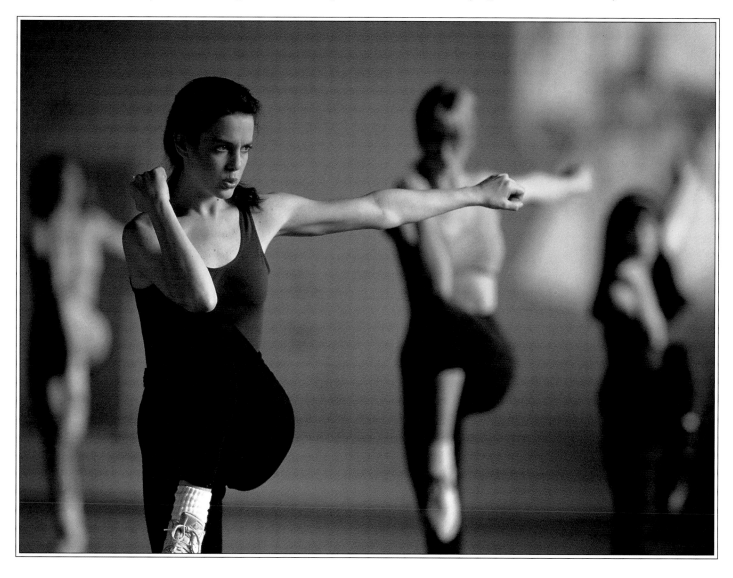

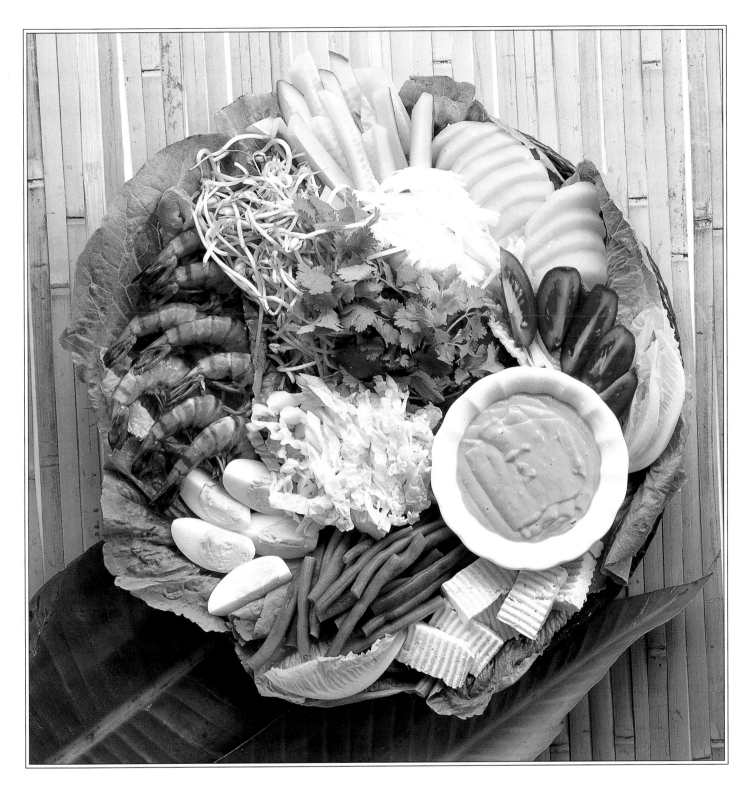

ABOVE: A healthy diet is far from boring as long as you maintain variety and imagination in your food preparation.

along. In the first place, a healthy diet should be an enjoyable one. For conventional nutritionists, food intake is broken down into various essential ingredients, such as carbohydrates, protein, fats, vitamins and minerals; however, people generally do not think in this way but eat meals or snacks which are a mixture of various elements. What is useful is to have an understanding of which foods contain which of these ingredients, and then to look at the overall balance within the diet. Balance is probably the key word in nutrition, and it is the unbalanced nature of many Western diets that lowers vitality and may lead to ill-health. With a better understanding of the elements it is easier to create a healthy diet without too much thought and analysis.

CARBOHYDRATES

Carbohydrates are our main source of energy, and need really to form the major bulk of our diet. They are broken down in the body into glucose, and used immediately for energy or else converted into glycogen for short-term storage in the liver. An excess of carbohydrates over time will be changed and stored as fat. This is a particular danger with refined carbohydrates or sugars, which do not take much processing in the body and provide large amounts of instant energy. Since they have less starchy bulk, refined carbohydrates do not make you as full, and therefore it is easier to eat too much of them, leading to fat storage and obesity.

The main sources of unrefined carbohydrates, providing dietary fibre and trace elements, are flour and grains, beans, peas and lentils, and potatoes. With grains, this is especially true when they are unprocessed, like wholegrain bread, whole oat cereals, muesli, wholewheat pasta, brown rice and so on which supply long-term energy supplies. For more immediate energy, fresh fruit, dried fruit or vegetables such as carrots or beetroot are high in fructose, or fruit sugar. This is easily broken down by the body for energy use, and since fructose metabolism does not require insulin, it can be an essential energy resource for diabetics.

There is almost complete accord among official governmental nutrition advisers and natural dietary therapists, that carbohydrates should be the chief element in our diet. In practical terms that means eating plenty of fresh

BELOW: Eat plenty of bread, wholemeal or granary if possible.

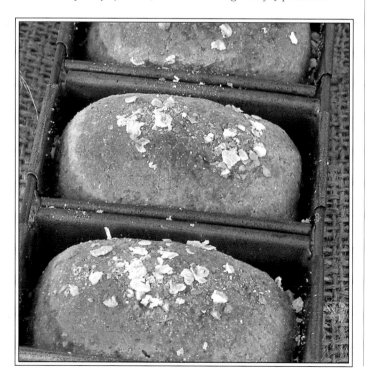

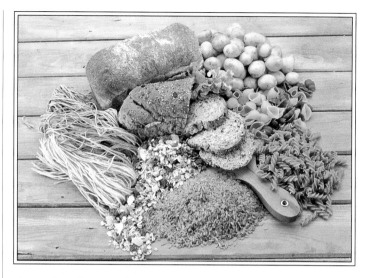

ABOVE: Bread, rice and pasta are important for the carbohydrates which give us vital energy.

vegetables and fruit, grains of all kinds (unless there are specific reasons for avoiding a particular grain, such as with a wheat allergy), potatoes, beans and lentils. A recent piece of advice from official organizations, for instance, has been to consume five portions of fruit or vegetables a day.

FIBRE FACTS

Fibre is important to a healthy diet. Your body cannot digest it, so, in rather basic terms, it goes in and comes out, taking other waste with it. Fibrous foods include bread, rice, cereals, vegetables, fruit, and nuts. We should aim for about 30g (just over 1oz) of fibre a day. These are some examples of good fibre sources.

GOOD SOURCES	AVERAGE PORTION	GRAMS OF FIBRE
wholemeal pasta	75g/3oz (uncooked)	9
baked beans	125g/4oz	8
frozen peas	75g/3oz	8
bran flakes	50g/2oz	7
muesli	50g/2oz	4–5
raspberries	100g/3½oz	6
blackberries	100g/3½oz	6
banana	average fruit	3.5
baked jacket potato	150g/5oz	3.5
brown rice	50g/2oz	3
cabbage	100g/3½oz	3
red kidney beans	40g/1½oz	3
wholemeal bread	1 large slice	3
high-fibre white bread	1 large slice	2
stewed prunes	6 fruit	2

PROTEINS

Proteins are the essential body-builders, helping us to create muscles, bones, tendons, hair, skin and nails. They are also vital in most of our hormone and enzyme production. The first thing to say about protein is that in most developed countries people eat too much, so the problem is not so much increasing those foods that are high in protein but getting the balance right. An excess of high protein foods in the diet will be converted into glucose for energy use or else stored as fat.

Foods rich in protein include meat, fish, poultry, eggs, milk and other dairy products, nuts and seeds, beans and lentils, and grains (bread has a little under ten per cent protein). Human protein is made from a number of simple substances called amino-acids, and these need to be present in certain amounts or combinations in the protein in our diet for us to make use of them. Animal sources do contain the right amounts of these amino-acids, but also contain relatively high levels of fat. Plant sources of proteins often need to be combined in order to give adequate levels of amino-acids; this can be something as simple as beans on toast, or a spicy bean dish with rice, and generally means having a more varied, or even a more adventurous diet.

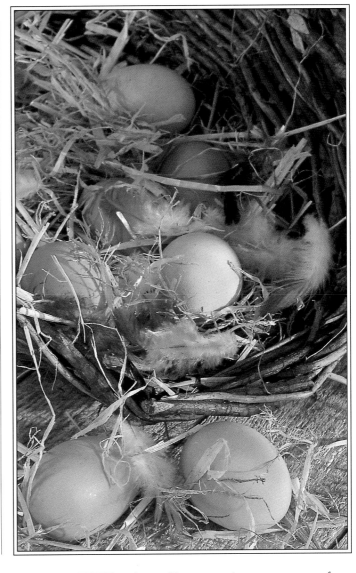

LEFT: *Dairy products, such as milk, butter and cheese, supply us with not only protein but also fat.*

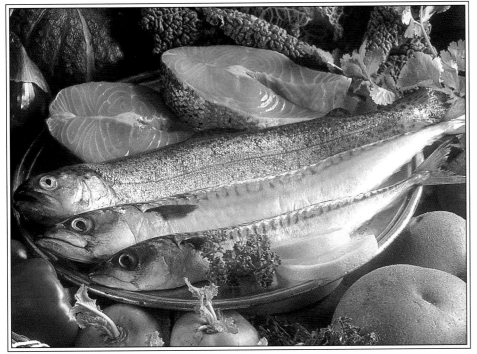

ABOVE: *Eggs are an important source of vitamins and protein but you should not eat more than two to three a week.*

LEFT: *One of the best sources of protein, fish is high in vitamins and minerals and is highly recommended by nutritionists.*

BELOW: *Eat unsalted nuts for their protein.*

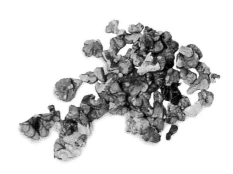

FATS

Fats are vital too, helping to form part of the cell structure and maintaining our inner organs and nerves. They also act to provide insulation and temperature regulation. It is, however, well-recognized that in the developed world much of our diet is too rich in fats, especially animal fats, and this is a major factor in heart disease, obesity and even some cancers, especially when we have such sedentary lives. Growing children, however, especially active ones, do need fats more than adults, and we should not reduce their intake so much.

Advice on fat-containing foods tends to be what to reduce rather than what to increase. Meat and dairy products can contain concentrated sources – a nice, juicy steak may have 30 per cent fat, for example. There are some differences between the effects of saturated fats (from animal products) and unsaturated fats such as are found in oily fish like salmon or plant oils like sunflower products. In general terms, move the emphasis towards the latter, using oils such as olive, sunflower, corn or safflower with salads or in cooking, but most people need to reduce all kinds of fats; they are the most concentrated sources of energy and anything over small amounts easily leads to obesity. There are plenty of reduced-fat items, particularly dairy products, which are now available and which can help in controlling fat intake.

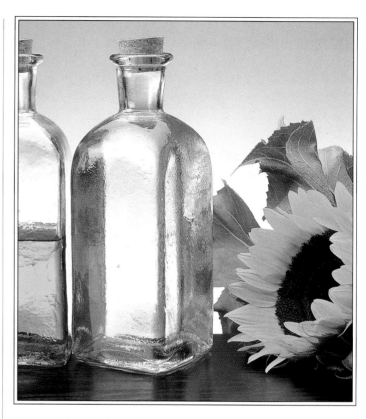

ABOVE: Oil made from the seeds of sunflowers is an unsaturated fat which should be used instead of animal fats in cooking. Avoid frying foods, however, and grill or steam instead.

EASY WAYS TO CUT DOWN FAT AND SATURATED FAT

EAT LESS	INSTEAD
Butter and hard fats.	Spread butter more thinly, or replace it with a low fat spread or polyunsaturated margarine.
Fatty meats and high fat products such as pies and sausages.	Buy the leanest cuts of meat you can afford and choose low fat meats like skinless chicken or turkey. Look for reduced-fat sausages and meat products. Eat fish more often, especially oily fish.
Full-fat dairy products like cream, butter, hard margarine, milk and hard cheeses.	Choose skimmed or semi-skimmed milk and milk products and try low-fat yogurt, low-fat fromage frais and lower fat cheeses such as skimmed milk soft cheese, reduced-fat Cheddar, mozzarella or Brie.
Hard cooking fats such as lard or hard margarine.	Choose mono-unsaturated or polyunsaturated oils for cooking, such as olive, sunflower, corn or soya oil.
Rich salad dressings like mayonnaise or salad cream.	Make salad dressings with low-fat yogurt or fromage frais, or use a healthy oil such as olive oil.
Fried foods.	Grill, microwave, steam or bake when possible. Roast meats on a rack. Fill up on starchy foods like pasta, rice and couscous. Choose jacket or boiled potatoes, not chips.
Added fat in cooking.	Use heavy-based or non-stick pans so you can cook with little or no added fat.
High-fat snacks such as crisps, chocolate, cakes, pastries and biscuits.	Choose fresh or dried fruit, breadsticks or vegetable sticks. Make your own low-fat cakes and bakes.

VITAMINS AND MINERALS

Vitamins and minerals are needed for proper growth and development and body maintenance. They control the absorption of other nutrients and without them a series of complaints can develop, from headaches to sterility. There are 13 major vitamins which, apart from K and D, must be obtained from the food we eat. The fresher the food the higher its vitamin content. Food loses its vitamins through cooking, exposure to light or cold and storage, so buy small quantities of fresh food and eat it as soon as possible.

RIGHT: Supplements are an important source of vitamins but do not rely on them for all your requirements.

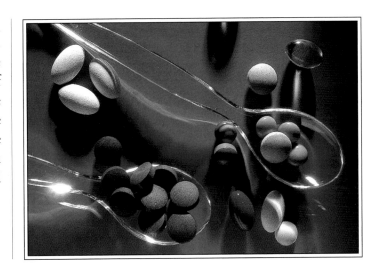

MINERAL AND VITAMIN VALUES		
VITAMIN	**SOURCES INCLUDE**	**BENEFITS**
Vitamin A	Liver (especially fish livers), egg yolk, fortified margarine, oily fish, oranges, apricots, carrots, tomatoes, melons, dark green leafy vegetables.	Eyesight; skin; may protect against cancer.
Vitamin B1	Most foods – including wheatgerm and pulses, wholegrains, brewer's yeast, nuts, fortified breakfast cereals.	Helps break down carbohydrates; nervous system; repairs body tissues.
Vitamin B2	Brewer's yeast, liver, kidney, dairy produce, wheat bran, wheatgerm, eggs.	
Vitamin B3	Wheatgerm, wholegrain cereals, meat, fish.	Essential for tissue chemical reactions.
Vitamin B6	Avocados, liver, wholegrains, egg yolk, lean meat, bananas, fish, potatoes.	Nervous system; skin; red blood cells.
Vitamin B12	Liver, kidney, some fish (including shellfish), eggs, milk.	Healthy blood and nerves.
Vitamin C	Citrus fruits, potatoes, tomatoes, leafy greens.	Helps heal wounds, may fight colds, flu and infections; protects gums, keeps joints and ligaments in good working order.
Vitamin D	Fish liver oils, fatty fish, eggs, fortified margarine, also synthesized by ultraviolet light.	Calcium deposits in bones.
Vitamin E	Vegetable oils, some vegetables, wheatgerm.	Cell growth; antioxidant.
Vitamin K	Most vegetables – especially leafy green ones, liver.	Essential in production of some proteins.
MINERAL	**SOURCES INCLUDE**	**ESSENTIAL FOR**
Calcium	Cheese, milk, yogurt, eggs, bread, nuts, pulses, fish with soft bones such as whitebait and tinned sardines, leafy green vegetables.	Healthy bones, teeth and nails; muscle and nerve function; blood clotting; milk production in nursing mothers.
Iron	Liver, red meat, oily fish, wholegrain cereals, leafy green vegetables.	Makes haemoglobin, the pigment in red bloods cells that helps transport oxygen around the body.

HEALTHY EATING

So, what advice can be given on foods? Our needs do vary throughout life, so there is no single diet that can be suggested – thank goodness! Children and teenagers need more protein, and most other nutrients, due to their growth rates, and pregnant women have an extra need too. Hard physical work or other activity increases demand, while older and less active people may require fewer calories. What we all need is varied, healthy and enjoyable food.

Three key words are freshness, wholeness and variety. As far as possible make fresh foods the major part of your food intake – fresh fruit and vegetables, freshly cooked bread, pasta or other grains, and a little freshly prepared meat, poultry, fish or other protein-containing foods. Preparation of foods should aim to retain as much of the original goodness as possible, so grill or bake foods rather than frying them. Wholeness can be taken to indicate not just trying to use wholegrains but cutting back on processed foods as far as possible. Try to have fresh foods first, then frozen and only occasionally resort to packaged or canned food. Variety means exactly that; it is as unhealthy to eat just oranges all day as it is to eat nothing but hamburgers all day.

BELOW: Take advantage of the many kinds of fruit available around the year, and vary your intake as much as possible.

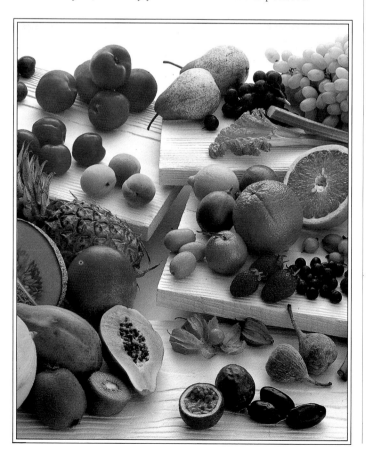

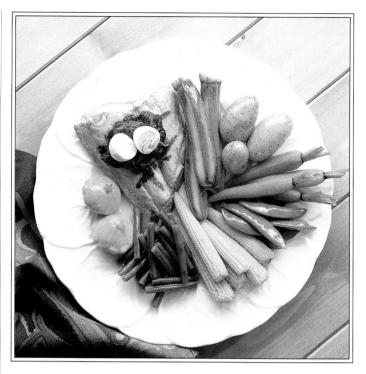

ABOVE: Steamed vegetables retain much of their vitamins as well as colour and flavour.

SOME IDEAS MIGHT INCLUDE:

❦ More fresh fruit and vegetables: they are high in vitamins and minerals and low in fats.

❦ Steadily increase fibre-rich foods, such as fruit, vegetables, wholegrains, beans and lentils.

❦ Eat fish, poultry and leaner cuts of meat, and avoid frying them as far as possible. Cut down on meat products such as pies, sausages and so on, which generally have high levels of fat.

❦ Eat fewer dairy products and use low-fat versions of, say, yogurt or milk.

❦ Keep pastries, cakes, biscuits and chocolates for special occasions.

❦ Drink plenty of water; many of us get dehydrated.

❦ Ease up on stimulants such as coffee and tea, and also alcohol.

❦ Try to use less salt – this also means reducing intake of processed foods, since they can often be high in salt.

❦ Enjoy food! There is a lot of pleasure to be gained from the taste and aroma of a varied diet.

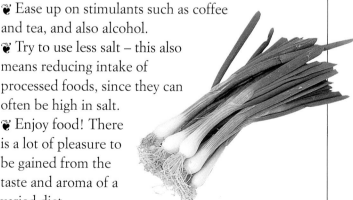

7-DAY HEALTHY EATING PLAN

This healthy eating plan gives suggestions for a balanced way of combining foods. Try to choose low-fat, low-sugar foods aiming to include plenty of wholegrain high fibre foods and 5-6 portions of fruit and vegetables each day.

To the suggestions below add your own choice of fruit juices and water and limited wine, tea and coffee. Try drinking some of the many blends of herb teas which are now available and which are a delicious, healthy substitute for tea and coffee. For snacks and desserts choose fresh fruit, and low fat fromage frais or yogurt with occasional high fibre bran muffins or carrot cake for treats.

RIGHT: Make sure the fruit and vegetables you buy are fresh and flavoursome, and buy little and often to gain full vitamin benefit.

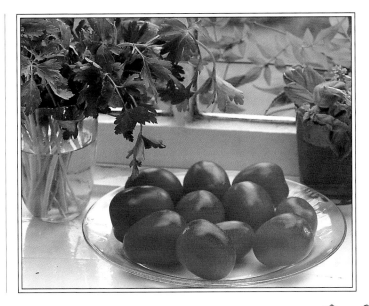

	BREAKFAST	LUNCH	DINNER
Monday	Fruit juice, porridge, fresh fruit.	Sardines or pilchards on toast.	Macaroni, cauliflower and broccoli cheese.
Tuesday	Grilled mushrooms or tomatoes on toast.	Homemade coleslaw with cottage cheese and rye crispbreads. Fresh fruit and oatbar or flapjack.	Salade Nicoise; lettuce, tomato, cucumber, new potatoes, tuna, olives, hard-boiled eggs, anchovies.
Wednesday	High energy drink, juice or milk, and banana, yogurt, honey and wheatgerm.	Onion soup with grilled cheese croutons. Fresh fruit and fruit cake.	Stir-fried vegetables and chicken or cashew nuts with rice or noodles.
Thursday	Muesli topped with low-fat live yogurt and chopped apple.	Wholemeal sandwich of cream cheese, avocado and salad. Fruit.	Pasta with tomato, bacon and mushroom sauce and parmesan cheese and mixed salad.
Friday	Fruit juice, cereal, toast and honey and fresh fruit	Hummous with crudites and wholemeal pitta bread or rye crackers.	Paella or risotto and green salad.
Saturday	Boiled, poached or scrambled egg on granary toast.	Jacket potato with baked beans and grated cheese, salad. Fresh fruit.	Grilled fish with fresh tomato sauce, steamed vegetables and new potatoes
Sunday	Fresh or soaked dried fruits with low-fat live yogurt. Wholemeal or granary toast.	Roast chicken joint with roast Mediterranean vegetables; whole garlic, peppers, courgette, aubergine etc, and potatoes or rice. Fruit and yogurt brulée.	Thick vegetable and lentil soup with wholemeal bread. Fresh fruit salad and cheese.

MOVE TO KEEP ALIVE

As far as exercise is concerned, the best phrase to sum up the importance of movement to your body and health is, "Use it or lose it". Inactivity, a sedentary lifestyle, means that our bodies steadily deteriorate and various health problems start to develop. Equally importantly, exercise helps to reduce the effects of stress and worry, and makes us feel better. The value of exercise is high at all times of life, for children growing up and developing strong bones and muscles, for adults to keep fit, active and healthy, and for older people to reduce problems like osteoporosis and simply to keep mobile and independent.

This is another area where official encouragement has occurred in recent years, with suggestions of a minimum of 20 minutes of brisk exercise three times a week as one example. Having activity goals can be very useful, but they should not act as a deterrent to getting started; any amount of exercise is better than none. It must be said, of course, that sudden, unaccustomed or inappropriate exercise can cause musculoskeletal problems, and people with certain conditions may need to seek medical advice before undertaking

BELOW: Exercise in the fresh air as much as you can with walks and cycle rides in the country.

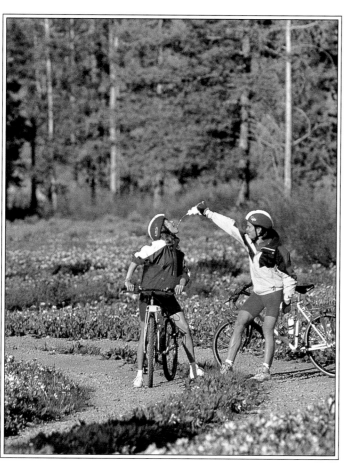

RIGHT: Take small amounts of regular exercise.

exercise. Nevertheless, steadily increasing exercise is likely to benefit the great majority of us, improving the efficiency of our heart, lungs and muscles, improving our posture and making us feel fitter and look healthier.

The first advice is to take the kinds of exercise that you enjoy and that you can incorporate into your lifestyle. Walking up and down stairs rather than taking the lift can be a simple example of fitting more movement into your life. Weekend walks, gardening, cycling or dancing are some leisure activities that can also help you to get fitter.

If you have not done much exercise for some time, do try to warm up and loosen the body before doing anything more strenuous, and don't exercise straight after meals. If you are ill or very tired, then limit physical exertion too. To allow easier movement, try to wear loose, comfortable clothing when exercising, and use the correct shoes and clothing when playing a particular sport. A good idea may be to join a class; with exercise like aerobics, low-impact exercises or weight-training, a class is essential to make sure that you are doing the movements safely and correctly. Personal trainers can provide detailed exercise programmes for you, with advice on the training zone, or optimal heart-rate, that you should aim for. Serious exercisers have access nowadays to all kinds of scientific back-up on how to plan and carry out exercise, but for most people it is most important to get fun and enjoyment out of physical activity.

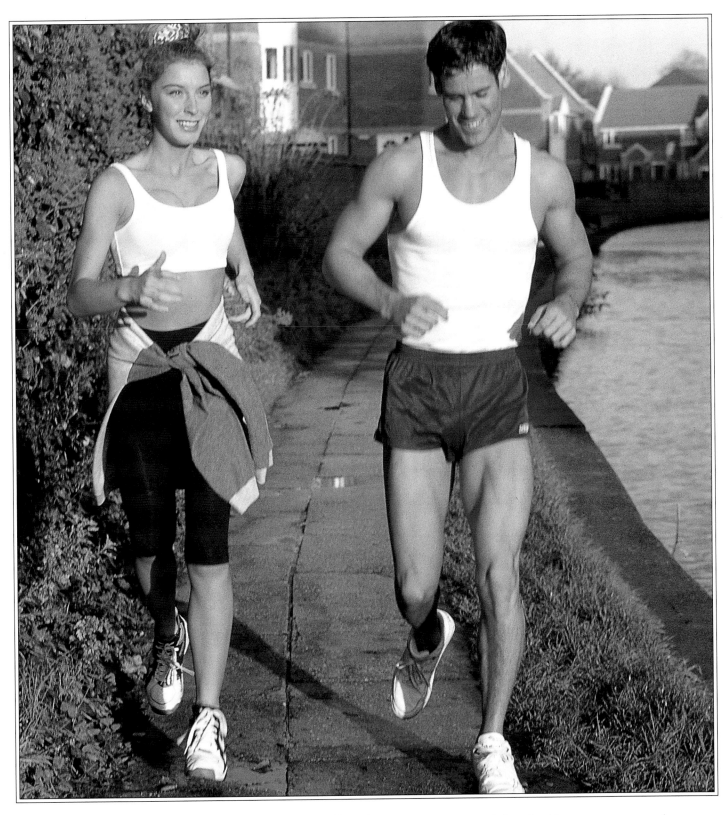

ABOVE: Exercising with friends adds encouragement and company.

Another important aspect of physical fitness is the effect it has on the way we feel about ourselves. Without becoming neurotic about your size and weight, try to take an interest in the state your body is in. An enjoyable and invigorating fitness regime, at a level you can sustain without undue stress, can enhance your mental and physical well-being. When you are unfit you tend to feel more lethargic and uninterested in the world and the people around you. A straight back, a spring in your walk and an alert, energetic expression will create a better impression than bad posture, slumped shoulders and uncoordinated movements. So improve your fitness and your self-esteem at the same time.

SHOULDER AND NECK EXERCISES

WARMING-UP EXERCISES

Some suggestions for warming-up exercises are given here. If you haven't done much exercise for a long time, or are recovering from a long illness, initially they may be enough on their own to get you more mobile. They will also be helpful to prepare you for something more strenuous. If you are exercising for the first time in a long while, pay attention to how your body responds. If you become out of breath or your heart races, stop, and ask your doctor's advice on suitable exercise. If you are more used to exercise, use this routine as a warm-up before moving on to something more strenuous. Try to breathe freely and comfortably when doing these and any other exercises, and remain aware of your body's responses to the movements.

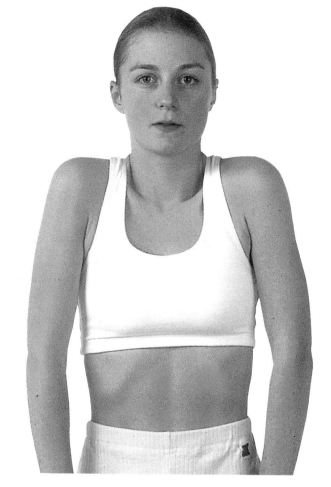

1 To loosen the shoulders and ease neck tension, try slowly rolling your shoulders in a circle, lifting them right up as they move round, and then dropping them down again.

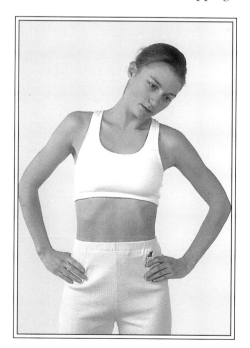

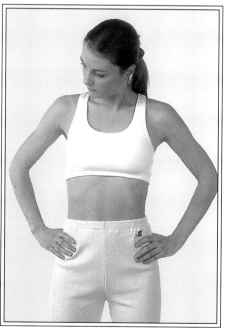

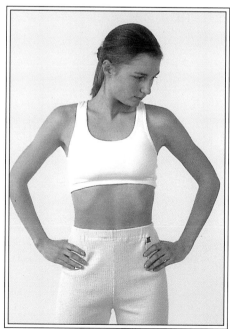

2 Stretch the neck muscles by dropping your head to the side, towards one shoulder and then the other, repeating three or four times.

3 Then slowly swing your head in an arc, from one side across your chest to the other side.

4 Repeat the swing three or four times, keeping control of the movement all the time.

ARM AND ABDOMEN EXERCISES

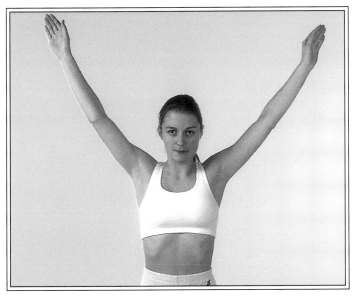

1 Swing your arms forwards in large circles, to begin to loosen the shoulder joints .

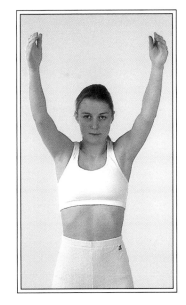

2 Then reverse the action and swing your arms backwards in large circles to open up the chest.

3 Facing forwards, twist your arms from one side to the other, letting them move loosely.

4 Continue the movement but begin to allow your head and trunk to move sideways with the arm swings.

5 Continue to twist right round, keeping your head in line with your arm movements.

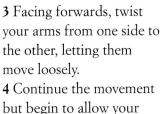

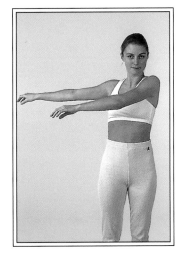

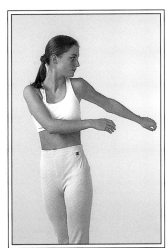

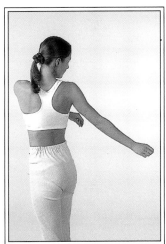

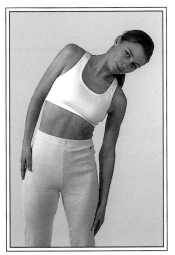

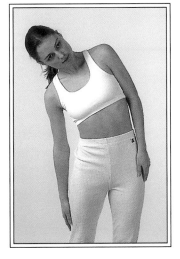

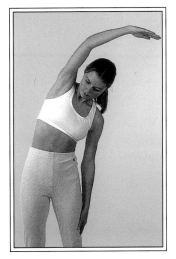

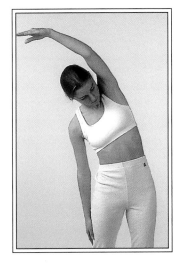

6 Bend sideways from the waist, keeping your hips still and moving your hand down towards your knee.

7 Return to an upright position, then bend to the other side. Keep your feet firmly on the ground.

8 Extend this movement into a bigger stretch by raising one arm in the air and bending sideways.

9 Repeat the movement in the opposite direction.

BENDING AND SQUATTING

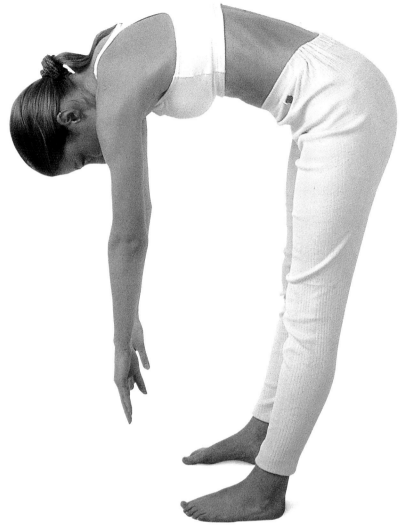

1 With legs about shoulder-width apart, bend forwards as far as you can, keeping your legs straight.

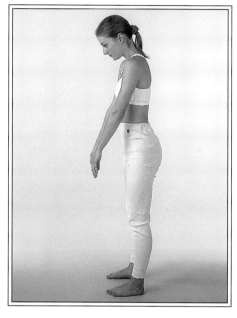

2 Steadily return to the upright. Repeat the action. If this is difficult, keep the legs slightly bent when bending forward, and gradually work on straightening the legs while you are leaning forward.

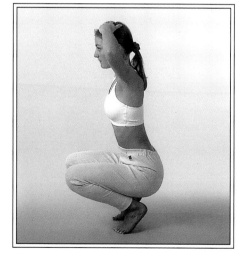

3 With hands on your head or hips, squat down, keep your back straight.

4 Come back to a standing position, returning to your tiptoes as you do so. Repeat the exercise serveral times.

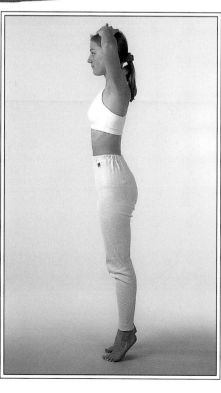

5 Try jogging, running or jumping on the spot. If you suffer from any back problems, you may be better off with a rebounder or using a step to go up and down to reduce impact – get professional advice if you are unsure.

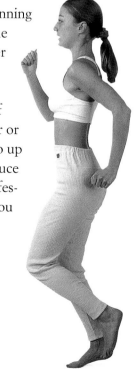

FLOOR EXERCISES

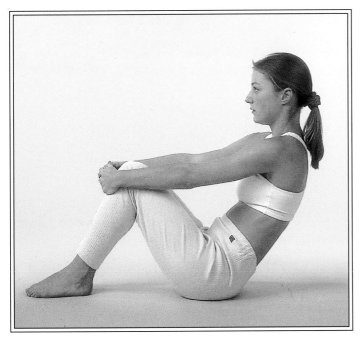

1 To tone and strengthen the abdominal muscles, try sitting on the floor, with knees bent and hands clasped around the knees. Lean back as far as comfortable, using your arms to support your weight, breathing out as you do so and holding for five seconds if possible.

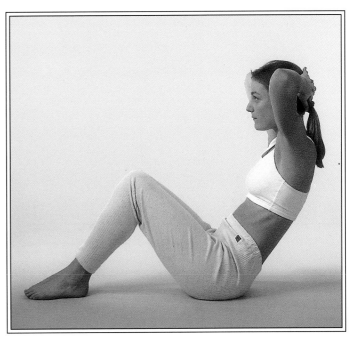

2 Repeat at least five times. As your muscles improve, try placing your hands behind your neck, so that the abdominal muscles do more work.

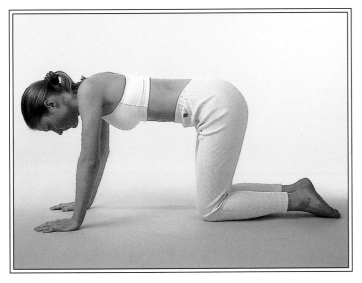

3 Go on all fours on the floor, making sure your hands are directly below your shoulders, and your knees are in line with your hips. Keep your back and neck in a straight line.

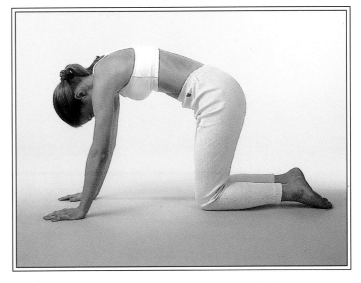

4 Then stretch and arch your back upwards, dropping your head down, hold this position for a few seconds, then return to the first position. Repeat several times.

You may use these exercises before harder physical activity, and/or as a cooling-down period after strenuous exercise, or simply on their own if you have a very sedentary life. If you have any pain or discomfort, then you may need to get advice – the old slogan "no pain, no gain" has been sidelined by more positive attitudes to movement. If you find you prefer doing exercises with others, to music or even while singing along yourself, then do so and have fun.

HYDROTHERAPY

Hydrotherapy, or the use of water for healing purposes, has an ancient pedigree, and different applications of using water can be found in many classical civilizations. Both the ancient Greeks and Romans used hot- and cold-water baths extensively, and many of the modern spas throughout Europe owe their origins to Roman bathing centres. Similarly, the Native Americans were familiar with the use of sweat-lodges, for physical and spiritual cleansing, and were proficient in various hydrotherapeutic techniques.

In recent centuries, however, some of this knowledge and expertise was lost. The therapeutic uses of water were largely revived in Europe in the nineteenth century by a Bavarian Dominican monk, Sebastian Kneipp. He believed that people had considerable innate healing powers and that water applications were a medium for stimulating, or occasionally soothing, our recuperative efforts. His ideas have continued to be influential to this day, and in spas in Germany it is possible to experience one of 50 or so different water applications for a variety of ailments.

Typical treatments may include contrast bathing, using alternating baths of hot and cold water. These are usually what are termed sitz baths, a kind of hip bath that immerses the lower trunk, while the feet may be placed in foot-baths of contrasting temperature in order to stimulate the circulation. Other forms of treatment may include high-pressure hosing with cold water, hot or cold body wraps, friction rubs, or baths with various ingredients added for extra elimination – for example, mud baths, Epsom salts baths or thalassotherapy (seawater baths).

Cold body wraps are made by soaking a sheet in cold water and wrapping

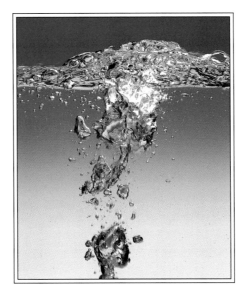

ABOVE: Fresh bubbling water is full of power and energy.

it around the body, then covering this with a dry sheet and blanket. The initial cold is quite quickly replaced by warmth. These wraps are used for a number of conditions such as chronic muscle strains and backache. The sitz baths are often recommended for conditions such as chronic constipation, congestion in the pelvic area, recurrent cystitis and period pains. The sprays have similar effects to the baths, depending on their temperature, but are generally more stimulating to the circulation. A milder effect is achieved by whirlpool baths, which are increasingly popular in homes, gyms and spas.

Some recent medical research has shown the benefits of cool baths for reducing high blood pressure and improving peripheral circulation, and the contrasting applications of hot and cold water compresses and such like have a strong effect on the immune system, so hydrotherapy has very definite physiological effects. As a note of caution, prolonged exposure to very hot water is not a good idea for pregnant women or anyone with hypertension or heart disease, so be careful with saunas, Turkish baths, whirlpools and so on. Regular shorter sessions are often more beneficial.

Home applications can be very simple; a sprained ankle or similar injury with swelling needs a cold application initially, such as an ice pack or cold compress. After a while, older injuries may respond to hot, then cold applications, while chronic areas of muscular stiffness often do better with just warm water treatments. Although largely neglected by orthodox medicine in the UK, European countries and indeed the US have been much more positive about hydrotherapy, and new research is confirming its potential.

BELOW: A soothing foot-bath will help everyday aches and stiffness.

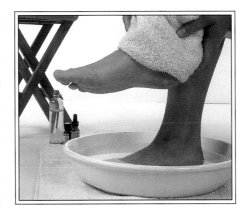

IRIDOLOGY

I ridology is the study of health and illness by diagnosing changes to the iris, or coloured part of the eye. The eyes have always been considered of some importance as indicators of internal health, or ill-health, but iridology as a distinct system dates back to the nineteenth century, to a Hungarian doctor called Ignatz von Peczely. As a boy, von Peczely had cared for an owl that had broken a wing. As the wing mended, he noticed that a thin black line which he had observed in the bird's iris gradually faded to little marks around a small dot. As an adult and a physician, von Peczely became more and more convinced through observation of his patients that similar illnesses produced similar changes and patterns of markings in their irises.

He published his findings in 1881, and they caused much interest throughout European and later American medical circles. In the 1950s in the US, Dr Bernard Jensen produced a detailed chart of the iris, locating each organ in the body to a specific part of the iris. His mapping system is quite complex, with various rings or zones relating to different systems, such as digestive, circulatory, lymphatic, muscular, skeletal and so on. Overall, the left eye shows up problems on the left side of the body, and the right eye the right side, although many disturbances seem to produce changes in both irises.

The map that Jensen and others developed divides the iris

BELOW: *Map of the eye showing which part relates to which part of the body.*

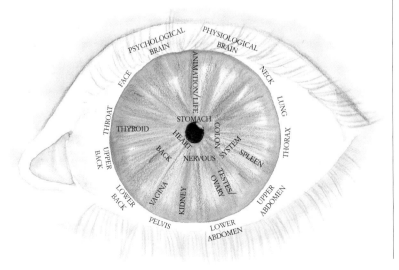

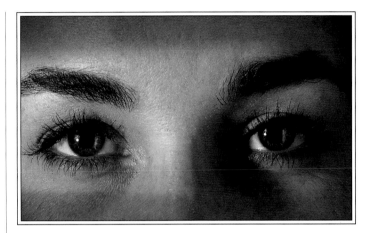

ABOVE: *A healthy eye will be clear, with no signs of inflammation, soreness or discolouration.*

into various sections, rather like a wheel divided by spokes. In each segment any markings within the iris are thought to be linked to different parts of the body, or else varying functions. Overlapping these divisions are the concentric rings mentioned above, which radiate from the centre of the eye outwards and are believed to show disturbances in the stomach, the glands and inner organs, the muscles and skeleton, and finally the skin and eliminative processes.

In the last 30 years or so, the knowledge of what an iris is able to show has increased, and a lot of work has been done on its complexity. There are some different schools of thought among iridologists and, in the main, although doctors find the general appearance of the eye – yellowing, dullness or unnatural brilliance, for example – an indication of ill health, conventional medicine dismisses completely the concept of specific, detailed links between parts of the body and markings in parts of the iris. Nevertheless, iridology has steadily grown in popularity among a number of therapists, who will use the technique as one of their diagnostic methods and as a non-invasive way of checking out internal functioning. An iridologist will diagnose rather than treat, and if any signs of degeneration, malignancy or disease are detected, patients are advised to see their GP.

Although many natural therapists are themselves sceptical of some of the claims of iridology, it is an area for fruitful research – our eyes are, after all, windows to the soul.

STRESS-MANAGEMENT

It is probably fair to say that the greatest threat to our health today, at least in the developed countries, is having more stress than we are able to handle. The increasing pace of lifestyles, the complexity of many professions, not to mention changes and added strains in relationships due to greater mobility and thus distance from others, has placed considerable burdens on our stress-management systems.

Nearly all natural therapies place great importance on stress as a probable factor in ill-health, and yet people need a certain amount of stress in order to become motivated and develop; so what is the problem? Our internal stress-coping mechanisms originally developed to cope with potentially life-threatening situations, the so-called "fight or flight" adaptation. However, these biochemical changes are all too often brought into play by other factors nowadays, from meeting deadlines or work crises to receiving the latest bill. When the body is placed in an almost constant state of alert, the adrenal glands become tired eventually and people are depleted and panicky rather than stimulated and awake.

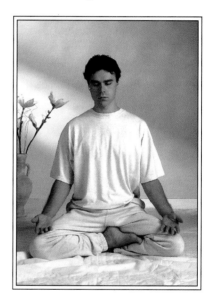

These problems have been recognized for a long time, and most natural therapies will offer some help with stress-related problems; in this section the focus is on some approaches which specialize in helping with stress-management directly.

ABOVE: Meditation is a well-known method for diffusing stress and tension.

OPPOSITE: Take time to relax and allow your body to rest during busy periods of life.

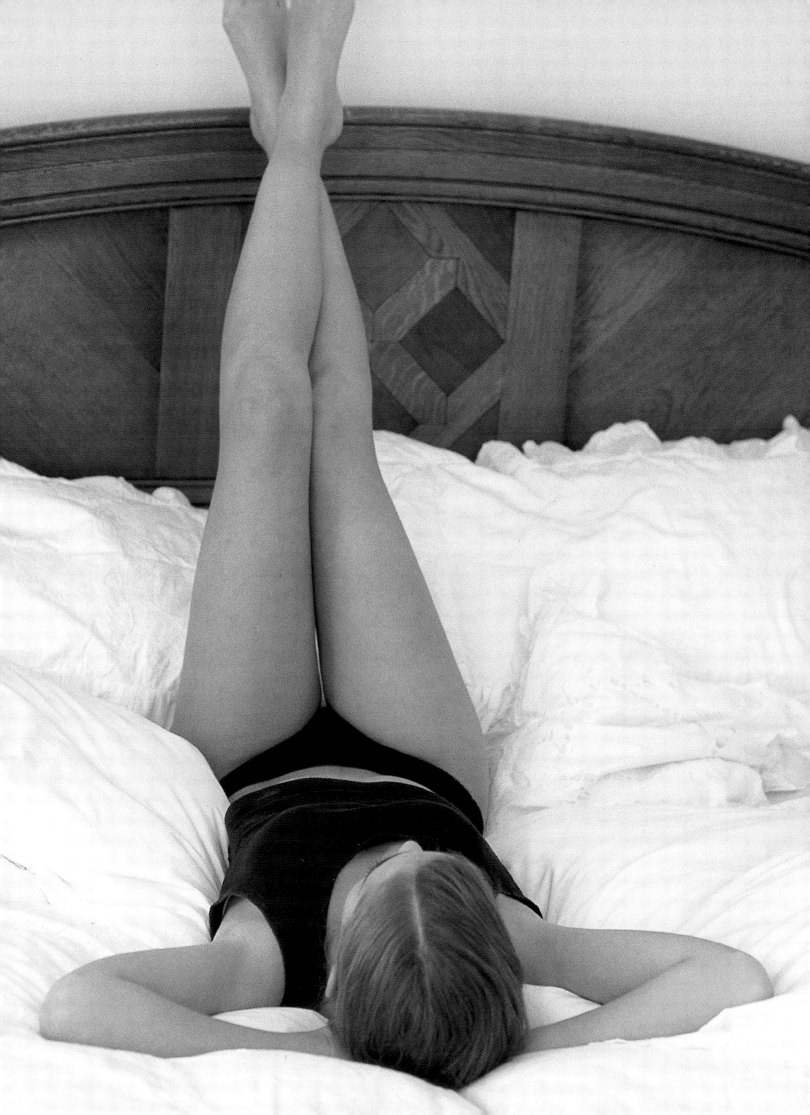

HYPNOTHERAPY

A person in hypnosis is not "asleep"; indeed they are often more aware of what is taking place than normal. Anybody (with a very few exceptions) can enter this deeply relaxed state, and indeed will, naturally.

It is believed that the state of hypnosis was used in ancient Egypt, South East Asia, and the Pacific island cultures. The hypnotic state is described in Greek and Roman writings too. The advent of Christianity appears to have marked the decline in its use, as it was then classed as witchcraft. It was, strangely enough, a Roman Catholic priest, Father Gassner, who in the late 1700s renewed public interest by using hypnotic inductions as a means of "casting out devils". Around the same time Anton Mesmer began to theorize about "animal magnetism", and the use of this phenomenon for medical purposes. He believed that Gassner was magnetizing his clients with the metal crucifix which he held. Mesmer attracted a lot of

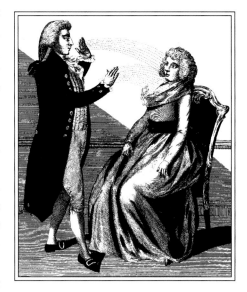

ABOVE: Mesmerism: an operator and his patient from E. Sibly's A Key to Physic and the Occult Sciences*, London.*

attention in France, and was later investigated by the French government and denounced as a fraud. It was left to James Braid to investigate further in 1841, and he is responsible for renaming mesmerism as hypnosis, from the Greek word *hypnos* meaning sleep, later trying to rename it mono-idealism, as he recognized it was not sleep but a concentration of the mind upon one channel of communication. But the words hypnosis and hypnotism had caught on, and change was impossible. Many more people after Braid developed theories about hypnosis and used it in the medical world. Perhaps the best-known exponent is a surgeon called Esdaile, who performed many serious operations painlessly using only hypnosis as an anaesthetic; some three hundred of these are carefully recorded. This method might well have continued had it not been for the discovery of chloroform and ether as chemical alternatives. It is interesting to note that hypnosis as anaesthetic is returning to popularity, especially in the US.

What then is hypnosis? It is a state of deep relaxation, a state of heightened awareness, combined with a feeling of calm lethargy. It can be best described as similar to that state between sleep and wakefulness when you are aware of your surroundings but unwilling to move. Its characteristics are a heightened susceptibility to beneficial suggestion and a much improved memory with access to "forgotten" or repressed memories stored in the unconscious mind.

In itself, the hypnotic state is very pleasant, but nothing more than that. It is very similar to the mental states achieved during meditation and yoga. It is what the therapist and client do together within this state that makes it therapy.

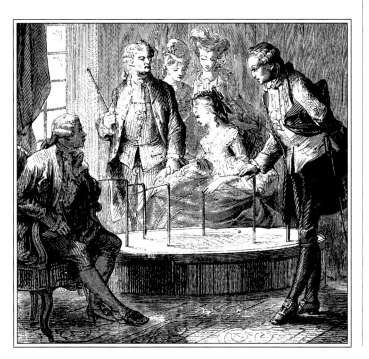

LEFT: Mesmer's tub at his consulting room in Paris which he opened soon after his treatise in 1779. The tub was a vat of dilute sulphuric acid and patients sat round it holding hands or holding on to one of the iron bars which projected from it.

SELF-HYPNOTIC INDUCTION

Self-hypnosis may not be suitable for anyone suffering from mental illness, or taking medication for a nervous condition. It is also potentially dangerous to use self-hypnosis to mask pain as this could lead to a serious illness going undetected. Ask your doctor's advice before using self-hypnosis in the above situations or if you have any doubts as to its suitability for you. It is also advisable to have one or more sessions with a properly qualified hypnotist to establish suitability and to receive instruction on how to use self-hypnosis.

Hypnosis as a natural state can be created in a number of ways, by audio, tactile or visual means. People can be shocked into hypnosis or coaxed or even bored into it. Self-hypnosis can be attained in many different ways too, but many therapists believe that by using the patterns outlined below, anyone can achieve a state of self-hypnosis. Initially, when learning these patterns, it may be useful to read them, slowly, on to a cassette tape, and then, preferably with headphones, use the tape to guide you into self-hypnosis. You may be reassured that should anything happen that requires your immediate attention, you will sit up straight away and deal with it as you would normally do: you are in control at all times. Non-intrusive music in the background can be helpful, too. Once you have learned to gain the state of hypnosis, you will be able to do so anywhere at any time that is useful to you.

STRESS MANAGEMENT

There follow three methods of self-hypnotic induction that can be highly beneficial to break a stressful day, to take five minutes to clear the mind before that important meeting, or just to unwind at the end of the day, so as to be clear thinking and able to enjoy the evening at leisure without carrying the worries of work into other areas of your life.

1 PHYSICAL RELAXATION

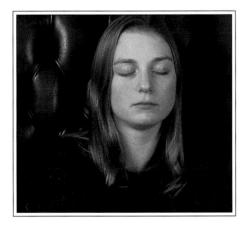 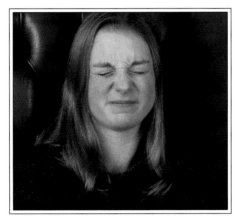 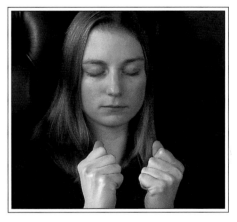

1 Settle back and relax in a chair or on a couch, or lie on your bed and just gaze upward, as if you were looking up through your eyebrows. Fix your gaze on a spot, either real or imaginary, and count down slowly from five to one. As you count down, imagine your eyelids becoming heavy, your eyes becoming tired, so that when you get to one, you can allow your eyes to close. Now begin to relax deeply. Think of the top of your head, your scalp, and concentrate on all the muscles, skin and nerve-endings there, deliberately relax them all and let go of all the tension.

2 Tense your facial muscles, scrunch them all up, around the eyes, the forehead, around the mouth, scowling and grimacing for a count of five seconds, and then release and let go, and feel that beautiful relaxation in all those muscle groups.

Thinking down through the neck and shoulder muscles and on into the tops of your arms, allow those muscles to sag down and become tension-free. Thinking over the muscles of the upper arms, tense those muscles for a count of five and let them go, let them relax down into the elbows and on to the forearms, just letting all those areas relax and let go.

3 Clench your fists, really tight, for a count of five, and release any tension, leaving the hands and arms heavy, easy and relaxed. With each breath you breathe out say to yourself, in your mind, the word "calm". Let any tension in the chest area drain away, as you think down into the stomach muscles, letting them relax too. Let all the muscles of your back relax. Thinking into your waist, your hips, and thigh muscles, let tensions drain away as you think down towards your knees … and on down into the shins and calves, allowing those muscles to relax, into the feet and toes, all muscles tension-free and feeling good.

2 THE STAIRS

Imagine a beautiful staircase stretching down in front of you made up of ten steps covered in a soft cream coloured carpet, perhaps lit with candles. Imagine you are standing on the tenth step up. Count backwards from 10 to 0, and as you count backwards, imagine each number as a step, and each step as a step down the staircase, into deeper and deeper levels of relaxation, so that by the time you get to 0, you can allow yourself to be as deeply relaxed as you can ever manage, while still aware of sounds around you.

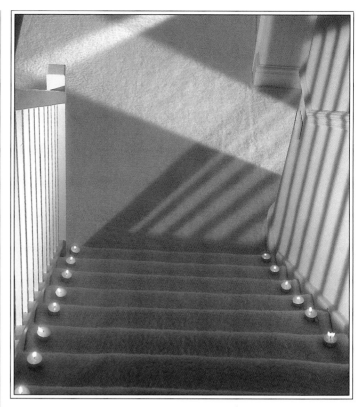

2. On step 6 you are becoming calmer … and calmer … even calmer still … Halfway down the stairs and you are continuing to relax, continuing to let go and feeling good. On step 4 you are relaxing even more … letting go … and by step 3 – sinking deeper … drifting further into this welcoming, relaxed state.

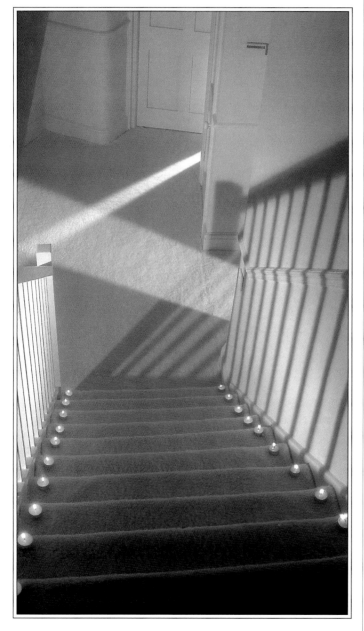

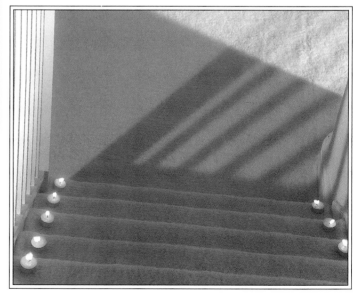

1 Imagine taking the first step down, relaxing and letting go. Take another step down, feeling beautifully at ease and at peace inside. On step 8 you are becoming more relaxed, and letting go even more … on 7 you are drifting deeper … and deeper … and even deeper down still …

3 On step 2, the last but one, you are enjoying those good feelings now, half-awake, half-asleep. By the time you reach step 1 you are nearly all the way down now, feeling beautifully relaxed. At the bottom of the staircase you are so beautifully relaxed, you can allow your mind to drift …

3 THE HAVEN

Allow your mind to drift … drift to a pleasant, peaceful place – a place that you know and where you can always feel able to relax completely. A safe, secure place where no one and nothing can bother you. It may be somewhere you have been on holiday, a beach or a place in the countryside. Or it may be a room you have had, one you do have or one you would like to have – an imaginary place. It's a place where you can always feel able to completely let go – a haven, a haven of tranquillity, unique and special to you.

In order to help you be in this place, notice first the lighting level. Is it bright, natural or dim, with any particular source of light – natural or manmade? Also notice the temperature level. Is it hot, warm or cool? Is there any particular source of heat? Be aware also of the colours that surround you. What are the shapes and textures and the familiar objects that make that place special?

Just be there, sitting, lying or reclining, enjoying the sounds, the smells and the atmosphere with no one wanting anything, needing anything, expecting or demanding anything from you. Now you can truly relax.

Now that you have reached that peaceful state of deep relaxation known as hypnosis, you can just relax and enjoy. You can bring yourself to full wakefulness at any time, by just slowly counting up from one to five, and allowing yourself to drift back to full physical and mental awareness, opening your eyes and getting on with the rest of your day, feeling restored and rested.

As with anything, the more you practise, the easier it will become, until you can shorten the patterns by just doing the following steps. You can achieve self-hypnosis in two to three minutes at most with these four steps.

1 Close your eyes.
2 Check that you are physically at ease.
3 Use the sound of the word "calm" with each breath you exhale.
4 Imagine yourself in your own "haven".

THE CALM TECHNIQUE

Once you have used the methods of self-hypnotic induction a few times, the mind has accepted the sound of the word "calm" as a signal for physical relaxation and mental calmness. This can then be used anywhere to control emotions and allow a return to clear thinking and just the right level of calm and relaxation for the situation. No one else will know you are doing it, but it puts you back in control. It is an ideal technique for a meeting that has become heated, and for immediately calming yourself before giving a presentation or having an interview.

BELOW: Your safe place might be a beautiful, sunlit woodland glade, with shafts of light illuminating the forest floor.

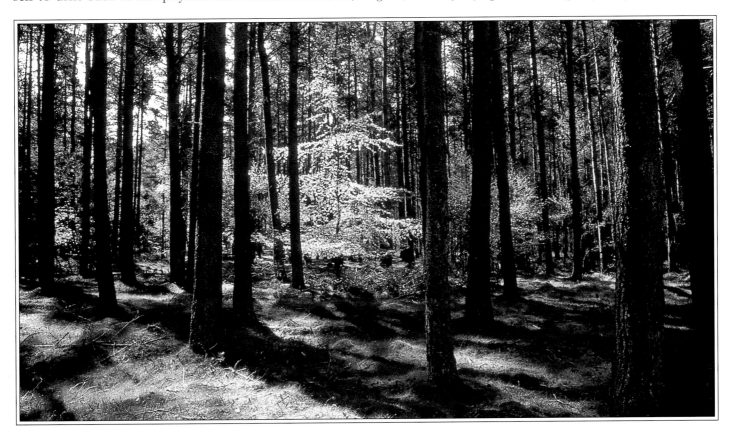

AFFIRMATIONS AND VISUALIZATION

Self-hypnosis can be usefully combined with affirmations, which have been brought into the forefront of psychotherapy in recent years. This deceptively simple device can be used by anyone and has proved remarkably effective.

It is recommended that you use this method while in self-hypnosis, having previously planned and memorized the affirmations involved. Thus you combine that ease of access to the unconscious mind and the effectiveness of repeated powerful positive phrases. You must say to yourself, out loud, a positive statement about yourself such as "I like my … (physical attribute);" "I am proud of my … (attitude or achievement);" "I love meeting people – they are fascinating;" or "I am quietly confident at meetings".

Notice the main points in these affirmations which can be used singly or together. They are in the present tense, and they are positively phrased and imply an emotional reward. You can create your own, and use them as often as you wish. The oldest and best-known affirmation is "every day in every way, I am getting better and better", written by Emile Coué at the end of the nineteenth century.

Yours is the most influential voice in your life, because you believe it. Used in this powerful combination, it can be truly effective in changing your expectations and reactions and in influencing outcomes.

In the same way that you can utilize your voice, so – and perhaps more powerfully – you can use your imagination. The imagination can stimulate emotions and can provide a direct communication with the unconscious part of the mind, and can also provide an impetus for registering new and more positive attitudes in the mind.

Visualization requires that you imagine yourself behaving, reacting and looking as you would wish to do in a given situation; for example a business meeting or a social gathering, and what that will mean for you. See your reactions, the reactions of those around you, and, most important, experience all the good feelings that will be there when this happens in reality. It is like playing a video of the event, on that screen on the inside of the forehead, the mind's eye, from the beginning of the situation through to the perfect outcome for you. Should any doubts or negative images creep into your "video", push them away and replace them with positive ones. Keep this realistic, and base it upon real information from your past.

Again the best time to do this is when relaxed mentally and physically – in self-hypnosis. Teach your mind to expect new, positive outcomes. This can be combined with affirmations and be doubly effective.

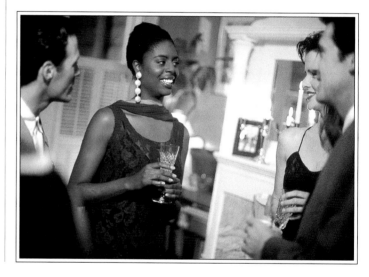

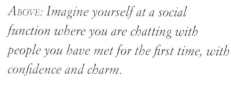

ABOVE: Imagine yourself at a social function where you are chatting with people you have met for the first time, with confidence and charm.

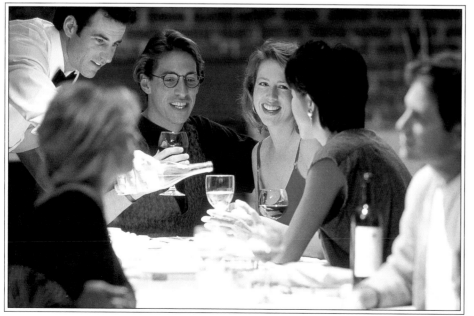

LEFT: Imagine yourself at a social gathering, such as a dinner party, where you are relaxed, comfortable and happy. You know that others are enjoying your company just as you are enjoying theirs.

THE SWISH TECHNIQUE

This technique is particularly useful to combat pre-interview or presentation jitters. It is a very effective method utilizing visualization and is derived from NLP (Neuro-Linguistic Programming), which is used throughout the world by therapists and patients alike. You can use this technique at any time when you feel relaxed. First thing in the morning, before getting out of bed, is a good time. Ideally, however, include this in your self-hypnosis programme and it will take just five minutes. Just work through it, with the instructions beside you, and then you will be able to do it on your own.

First, think of the event that is going to happen, an interview for example, about which you feel anxious. Focus in on that for a moment. You will probably find it much easier with your eyes closed.

Now create two pictures in your mind, filling the whole of the screen on the inside of your forehead, your mind's eye. The first picture is called "The Moment of Anxiety", and depicts the scene at the moment when you would expect to start feeling most anxious. Make the picture as detailed as you can: the room, the people, furnishings and so on – like a photograph you have taken yourself, so you are not in the picture, in full colour, detailed and brilliantly lit. When you are sure you have done that, put that picture to one side.

Next, form another picture; this one is called "The Moment of Achievement". This is a picture of you at the end of that occasion, looking really good, relaxed and happy, leaving the interview perhaps. Make this picture as detailed as you can: but most important of all – you, and the look on your face. The event has gone well and you feel really good. Make sure you have this in your mind as clearly as possible.

BELOW: The Moment of Anxiety.

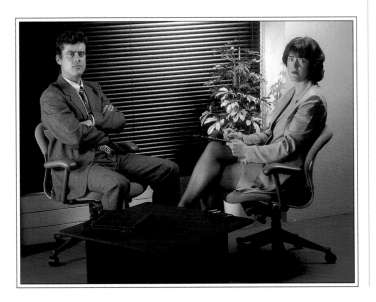

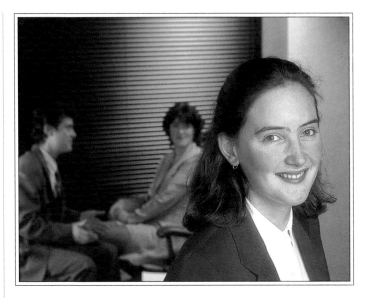

ABOVE: The Moment of Achievement.

Now see both of these pictures in the following way. The first picture, "The Moment of Anxiety", in full colour and brilliantly lit filling the whole of your mind's eye except for one of the lower corners, where, like a snapshot tucked into the frame of a larger picture, there is a small, dull black-and-white picture, "The Moment of Achievement".

When you have them clear and steady, swish them over – the small becoming large and full colour, the large becoming small and black and white. Allow yourself a few moments to really enjoy the feelings displayed on your face.

Clear your mind by opening your eyes and looking around you. Then set the pictures up again as they were before, with the Moment of Anxiety large and full colour and the Moment of Achievement as a small black and white snapshot, then swish them over. Do that exercise three more times, making five times in all.

Use the SWISH technique once a day for about a week before the situation you have in mind. You will find that very soon it is impossible for you to hold the first picture in your mind's eye without the second one automatically taking over. When this happens, you know that you have reprogrammed your mind for success rather than failure. Then repeat the exercise for two more groups of five to make absolutely sure.

It is under your control now. You can use this exercise to help yourself to gain the right attitudes so that you can be successful in many different situations.

Under no circumstances should the patterns illustrated here be used on someone else, nor should any effort be made to delve into personal history or past lives without the aid of a professional therapist. It can lead to situations that can quickly get outside of your competence.

MEDITATION

The word "meditation" means different things to different people. In the Western philosophic and religious tradition it can simply mean turning an idea or concept over in one's mind. What it has generally come to mean today is some form of clearing or emptying of the mind. A word such as "contemplation" may have been used at other times to mean the process of coming to a central point, focusing and quietening the mind. These practices are often referred to simply as "sitting".

Very often the word "meditation" is associated, in many people's minds, with all sorts of bizarre practices involving wearing long robes and sitting on the floor with your legs tied in a knot for hours on end. In short, there is a lot of mystification surrounding the idea of meditation. By describing some basic principles and aims in this chapter, and intro-

BELOW: When you are meditating make sure you are in a quiet, peaceful place with no risk of interruption or distraction.

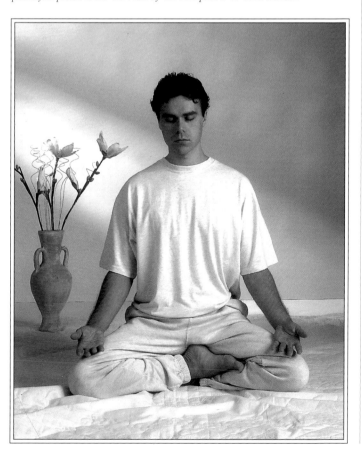

ducing some simple exercises which should benefit most people, some of that mystification should be dispelled.

There are hundreds of different schools of meditation, many associated with some form of religious practice, and many that are not. Some of these varied forms of meditation may include techniques such as complex visualizations or chanting words or sounds known as "mantras". Many of the world's great religions also make provision for retreat from the world in order to focus more closely on meditation for short or long periods. Practices of this kind have great value, but often form the basis for widely held and perhaps stereotyped ideas about what meditation involves. All of these techniques, and more, can also be practised without the necessity of being a follower of any particular religious tradition. (Incidentally, the exercises presented in this chapter are considered to be quite compatible with whatever religious belief, if any, an individual may already hold.)

Of course, you may choose to incorporate any, or all, of the above exercises into your practice, but none of them is strictly necessary in order to gain the benefits that meditation can bring to a modern, stressful lifestyle. Meditation is a truly holistic activity in that, ideally, the whole system of body, mind and spirit is involved and benefited.

BODY

The physical benefits of meditation are easily quantifiable and plenty of research documentation exists. These include relaxation, improvement of sleeping patterns, lowering high blood pressure, helping recovery from fatigue and a general beneficial effect on most stress-related disease. Posture can be helped, too, in that better posture leads to better meditation which in turn leads to better posture! The same can be said for relaxation. The mind cannot let go until the body relaxes, and vice versa.

Meditation is sometimes seen as a kind of vanishing upwards into rarefied heavenly atmospheres, rejecting all that is grossly physical. On the contrary, awareness of the body is an essential part of effective meditation. A kite can only fly if the string is firmly held on the ground. Many of the emotional stresses and upsets that people experience can be held as tensions in the body and therefore be fairly

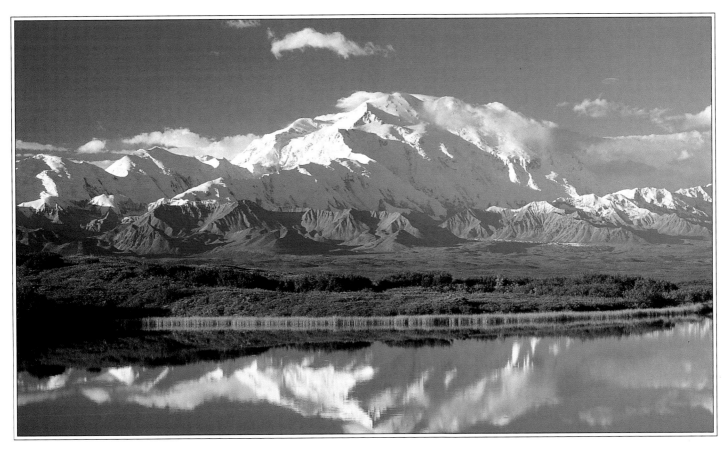

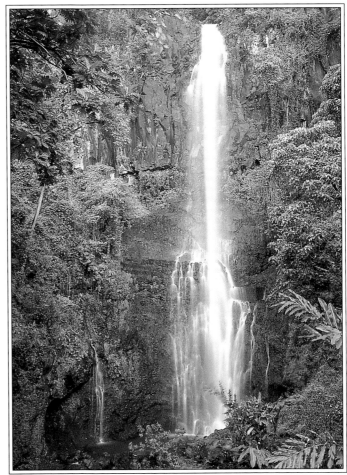

ABOVE AND RIGHT: A beautiful scene, such as mountains or a waterfall, can help evoke a feeling of wholeness, joy and peace. Use images such as this in your mind's eye when you are meditating. It may be a special place where you have been happy which holds personal significance for you, or it may be somewhere you have always dreamed of visiting which you have a strong mental picture of. Make the image in your mind as real as you can.

unconscious. Through the process of conscious relaxation of body and breathing that meditation entails, these stresses can be unlocked from their hiding places in the muscles and joints and simultaneously released. There was once a school of yogis in Tibet famous for their one principle or mantra: "Mind in the body, bum on the ground!" One can go a long way with a very simple awareness of body and breath.

Most traditions, both in the East and the West, agree that the body is bound together by a subtle form of energy (called *qi* in China, and a variety of names in other parts of the world) which manifests in forms known as the aura, acupuncture meridians or *chakras*. The increased sensitivity that develops from paying attention to natural bodily processes often results in a perception of this energy (perhaps as warmth, tingling, pressure, lightness or other such sensations). At this point the differentiation between mind and body begins to dissolve.

MIND

Meditation can improve the ability to concentrate, the ability to listen, both to others and yourself, and is a good way of monitoring the "internal weather". It is said that rates of depression and suicide are rising steadily in Western society and many commentators point to the breakdown of communities, people's divorce from the natural world and the poor living conditions of many. But if people cannot change their external conditions to any great degree, they can take responsibility for changing their attitudes and reactions – the way the mind interacts with the world. One of the safest and most effective ways to bring about this change is to meditate. People are able to be more self-sufficient and begin to let go of the addictions and dependencies they may have, such as drugs, food, television or sex, in which many seek refuge from reality. Paradoxically, meditation is not an escape from the real world; in fact it leads to a deeper engagement with, and awareness of, one's life in order to transform it.

The forms of meditation described in this chapter do not involve suppressing the thoughts or emotions with rigid self-control. What is required is more of a drawing together, paying ever closer attention, becoming absorbed in your object of meditation. If meditation is not a rejection of body, neither is it a rejection of mind – specifically of thoughts. Thinking is what the mind, or more accurately, the brain, is designed to do. This is its contribution to humankind's survival for the thousands of years we have been on this planet. In a way, trying to stop thinking would be like trying to stop breathing. What is even more important is to change one's attitude towards these thoughts, perhaps even the nature of them, not by rigid control but by developing what might be called a feeling of inner spaciousness that can include any thought or emotion. There is then less jostling for position, less anxiety and fewer demands for attention from one's thoughts.

Imagine a little girl, tugging at your sleeve persistently, determined to tell you something. You try to ignore her and perhaps even get angry, which then results in tears and uproar. If instead you turn round and give her your absolutely full attention, she may either suddenly become shy and run away, or whisper her few but terribly important words and then be satisfied to go and occupy herself elsewhere. Thoughts can behave in a very similar way. If your adult self is clear enough in its intention to meditate, the thoughts can continue with their play without causing disruption.

In a sense most people might be described as sleepwalking through life for all the engagement they have with it. The path of meditation offers a way of becoming more awake and alive to every aspect, inner and outer. The mind ceases to be a burden and distraction and instead becomes a tool for paying very good attention to the present moment. The practice known as "mindfulness" is simply carrying this present-centred attention into one's daily life and activities, whether walking, running or doing household chores. In this way meditation practice begins to become relevant to "real life" and not something separate and isolating.

RIGHT: Adopt a position which you feel at ease and relaxed in when you are meditating. Wear clothing which is loose and comfortable and which does not restrict you in any way. There is no correct way to sit, it is up to the individual to find a posture which suits them.

SPIRIT

The words "spirit" and "spirituality" can be very loaded for many of us with both negative and positive connotations. Those who may have suffered at the hands of dogmatic, judgemental or fundamentalist religion may feel understandably wary of this area and reject it altogether. However, spirituality may not necessarily have anything to do with any organized religion or philosophy. It need not even include the word "god". It might be useful to think of the word "spirit" in the context of phrases such as "in good spirits", "in the right spirit" or "a spirited horse".

Your spirituality is simply your relationship to whatever is most important or meaningful in your life – whatever nurtures you and fulfils your deepest needs. For some people this may be money, possessions or status, but going beyond these things, ask what it is they depend on and why you need them. You may not come up with any definitive answers, but it is the asking of the questions that is important. This inquiry may lead you to discover what is truly meaningful for you; perhaps loved ones, family, home, an appreciation of beauty, honesty, a desire to discover the true meaning of life.

WHEN AND WHERE?

How often should I practise? How should I sit? are questions often asked by those starting out on the path of meditation, once the basic exercises have been explored. For both these questions there are no "right" answers, no one "proper" way of meditating. Individuals explore for themselves, evolving an effective and appropriate practice.

As to frequency of practice, some schools suggest many hours a day, some advocate quality rather than quantity – a short, focused period of meditation of five or ten minutes. Regular practice is certainly helpful, preferably daily. Building a new habit into one's life may take time, but of course anything becomes easier with regular practice. Eventually, it may well feel indispensable. For some people self-discipline works well, although listening to the voice in your head which governs your discipline may be very interesting. Are you barking orders at yourself, judging yourself a lazy, useless slug if you cannot manage half an hour's meditation every day at 6.35 a.m. precisely? Or is the voice more of an invitation to participate in a restful exploration of your inner workings? Is there any sense of this five, ten or 20 minutes of your day being set aside gratefully as a gift to yourself? The greatest incentive known for doing anything is that it is enjoyable and makes one feel good. If meditation practice becomes as burdensome a necessity as, say, flossing your teeth or if it seems an indulgence that you do not have time for in your busy life, so full of important things to do, then you had better start examining your motives.

Sometimes being in a group or class to practise meditation can be very helpful. In a group one has the support of a roomful of people doing the same thing at the same time. A kind of synergy seems to exist in a group of people who are meditating together. Sometimes the reverse is true and solitude is what people need to get in touch with that single-pointed attention. Time, place and companions are all matters for individual choice and experimentation.

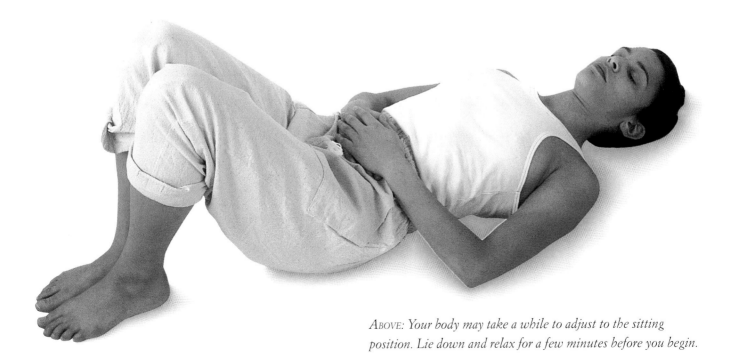

Above: Your body may take a while to adjust to the sitting position. Lie down and relax for a few minutes before you begin.

What about ways of sitting? Generally, meditation seems to work best when the spine is straight, but relaxed and vertical. The reasons for this are several. First, sitting upright is a very good way of staying awake and alert while the eyes are closed and the attention drawn inwards. If the body is upright, the breath can begin to move in and out freely and without obstruction. Also the muscles of the torso and spine have a chance to unknot themselves of old tensions. This may not always be an entirely pain-free process. Until the body becomes used to sitting in a new more conscious way, it may fight to be allowed back to its habitual "comfortable" state. These conflicts will pass, perhaps aided by some exercises such as yoga, tai chi or chi gung.

Eventually, proper posture will prove to be the most genuinely comfortable way of sitting still for a period of time. Sitting upright sends a message to the unconscious that although your eyes are closed, you are not going to sleep, as you would when lying down. On a more subtle level the body's *qi* energy, or life force, is able to move more freely if the spine is straight. Energy cannot move through tense muscles, so as relaxed a way of sitting needs to be found.

There is not necessarily any inherent virtue in sitting on the floor to meditate. Some people are very comfortable doing so, but if this is difficult for you, sitting in a chair is perfectly acceptable. Given the basic requirement of an upright spine, the way of arranging the legs is a matter for personal preference and respecting the body's limits. If sitting cross-legged on the floor, you will probably find it helpful to have a firm cushion at least 5–7.5cm (2–3in) thick under your bottom. This lifts the spine so that it is easier to sit upright. You may choose to kneel, in which case a larger cushion or a meditation bench under your bottom would be advisable to prevent cutting off circulation to the legs. If you feel most comfortable sitting in a chair, choose one that is the right height for you, or use some books under your feet. A firm, straight-backed chair is better than an armchair and if you can sit up unsupported, all the better.

A major objective in this discussion of posture is to ensure the free flow of breath through an open posture. Why is the breath so important in meditation? On the physical level, if the body is taking in enough breath, the brain then has sufficient oxygen to function at its peak and thus remain alert and focused. Breathing in by allowing the lower abdomen to expand enables the lungs to expand to their full extent and also relaxes the muscles of the torso and the internal organs. Many people breathe in a very shallow way, using only their shoulders and the top part of the chest. This way of breathing can produce stress and anxiety as it provokes the "flight-or-fight" response, meaning that rather than being alert in a relaxed and open way, they are tense and watchful. Breathing deeply, with the muscles of the abdomen relaxed, enables you to let go of deep levels of stress and tension, continuing and deepening the process of relaxation that begins with an aligned posture.

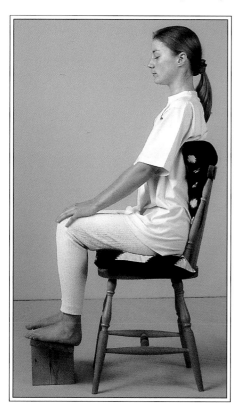

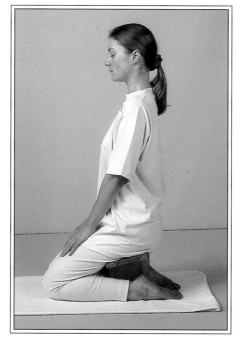

ABOVE AND LEFT: Choose your posture, sitting on a chair or kneeling on the floor.

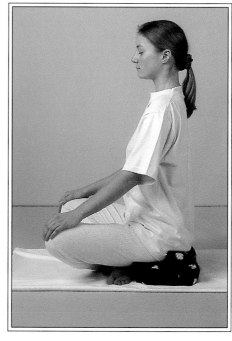

ABOVE: The traditional meditation position is sitting on the floor, with legs crossed.

FOCUSING

Your breath also provides an ever present and easily accessible focus for concentration. One is always breathing! Many schools of meditation teach focus on the breath in various ways. This may involve imagining that the breath originates in one particular point in the body. The points most usually focused on are the *hara* or *tan tien* – just below and behind the navel, or the heart – in the centre of the chest. The crown of the head, the base of the spine or the soles of the feet may all be included in the awareness. Focusing on the breath can also take the form of noticing the physical changes as the breath moves in and out, either at the nostrils or the abdomen. Meditation can be as simple as this, just breathing while sitting.

There are many ways of concentrating the mind in order to occupy that part of the mind that chatters incessantly, worrying and obsessing.

❧ Count the breaths from one to ten, then begin again.

❧ Notice the stillness at the changeover points at the end of the inhalation or the exhalation.

❧ Let an image arise that evokes a feeling of wholeness, joy and peace; perhaps a beautiful natural scene of mountains, the sea, a tree, the sun, a child or an inspirational figure and breathe this image into your heart.

FIVE MEDITATION STEPS

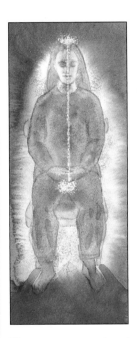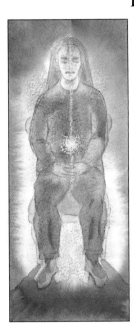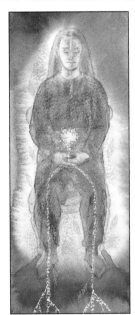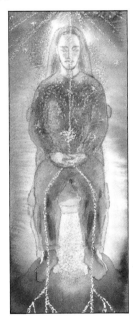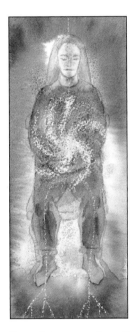

You can memorize these steps, have a friend read to you, or make a tape for yourself. Sitting comfortably but upright, feel your weight on the chair or cushion and relax into it. Imagine breathing in and out through your navel, taking a few deep breaths to settle in. Let your attention gather at a point at the base of your spine, imagine it as a point of energy. Notice what sensations you feel there.

1 Move your attention to the crown of the head, imagine a point of energy there. Notice what sensations you feel. Feel these two points align, connected by a line of light, inside the body near the spine. Allow energy to move freely between these two points.

2 Let your attention come to rest at a point of balance along this line, deep within you, at the centre of your being.

3 From this centre of your being, imagine the line of light extending downward through your legs and feet, relaxing the toes and sinking into the earth. Breathing out, let all tension and fatigue run down this line into the earth.

4 Breathing in, imagine drawing up, through the soles of your feet, fresh, transformed earth energy. Allow it to fill your whole body from the feet up to the crown of your head, bringing a feeling of being supported and cradled by the solidity of the earth. Return your attention and your breathing to the centre of your being. Imagine the line of light rising to the crown of your head and above, out into the clear blue sky, to the heavens. Breathe in fresh air.

5 Allow light and clearness from the heavens to radiate down the line of light to fill the whole body. Breathe into the centre of your being and feel the two energies, from the earth and the sky, mingling. From this centre let your attention be on your breath moving in and out (using one of the focuses suggested above).

PSYCHOTHERAPY

The basis of psychotherapy is the natural desire of someone with problems to want to talk to someone else about them, and it is often called the talking therapy. Practitioners generally refer to the people they see as clients rather than patients, to emphasize that it is not just for sick people but for anyone with problems. There are a number of schools of thought about the processes involved in psychotherapy, and the techniques range from simple supportive counselling to complex psychoanalytical theories about the underlying feelings behind current problems, and how to release them.

At its most basic level, psychotherapy is the creation of a space for somebody to air their problems in a caring, nonjudgemental and confidential atmosphere. This is almost an extension of a chat with a good friend, and the skill of the therapist lies not so much in what they might say, but in acting as a support for the client to unburden whatever is troubling the mind at the time. This kind of caring listening is often a part of the "treatment" given by many different skilled natural therapists.

Much of psychotherapy builds upon this passive listening, with somewhat more active interjections to point out areas of evasion, inconsistency or neglected issues. This helps people to break out of negative or destructive thought-patterns, to develop a better sense of their own identity, and to be happier in relationships.

Therapy can be short- or long-term. With relatively simple problems, for example, a phobia or single-issue problem, techniques such as behavioural or cognitive therapy may be used. These aim to change behaviour and attitude by respectively facing people with the feared experience or object, or getting them to try acting and thinking in a more positive way, in order to overcome the fear or anxiety. Such disciplines can be quite directive, with clients initially following instructions. Often, however, such apparently simple problems have deeper causes and a more long-term approach such as analysis may be beneficial.

Psychoanalysis is a distinctive, long-term approach, requiring a considerable period of training to become a practitioner, who therefore may be considered something of a specialist. The father of psychoanalysis was Sigmund Freud,

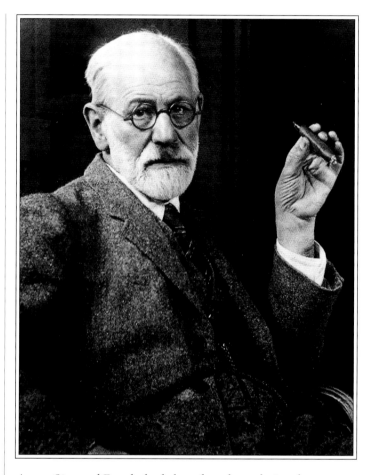

ABOVE: Sigmund Freud, the father of psychoanalysis, whose research revolutionized the way humans regard themselves.

the Austrian psychiatrist who developed theories of human experience that related psychological problems to our early childhood relationships with our parents. Dreams, fears and desires, both conscious and unconscious, and suppressed emotions are all investigated as factors in present problems. One of Freud's most brilliant pupils, Carl Jung, developed his own theories based upon archetypal symbols and myths, rather than childhood traumas, and numerous others have since added their own ideas to this complex field.

Thoughts and feelings are particularly significant in psychoanalysis, while other approaches also look at behaviour. Gestalt therapy, for instance, which was developed in the US by Fritz Perls in the 1950s, seeks to place a client's symptoms within the wider context of normal emotional responses; literally, the whole is greater than the sum of the parts. Changes in behaviour can affect feelings and thoughts, and vice versa. Trying to choose a suitable psychotherapist can therefore be something of a minefield for those who are unaware of the differences between the various schools. In the first place, decide how much change you want. Do you want to resolve a short-term problem, or undertake a complete overhaul of your attitudes and lifestyle?

Perhaps more than in any other therapy, the relationship between the client and the therapist is of great significance in psychotherapy and some time needs to elapse to build up confidence and rapport. Since people often gravitate towards therapies that suit their own personality, there can be a case for looking wider and experimenting a little – if you tend to be a thinker and good at intellectualizing problems, an approach that uses this technique may maintain this rather narrow view, so that a bodywork approach may be what you need; and vice versa of course.

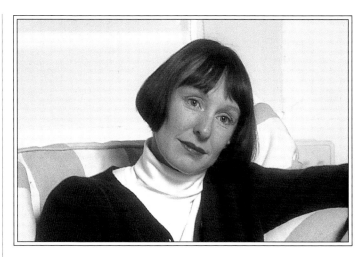

ABOVE AND BELOW: A psychotherapist will listen to what you have to say with a non-judgemental approach. Their detatched interest is very important, allowing you to explain feelings which would be difficult to express to friends or relations who are unable to maintain the same objectivity.

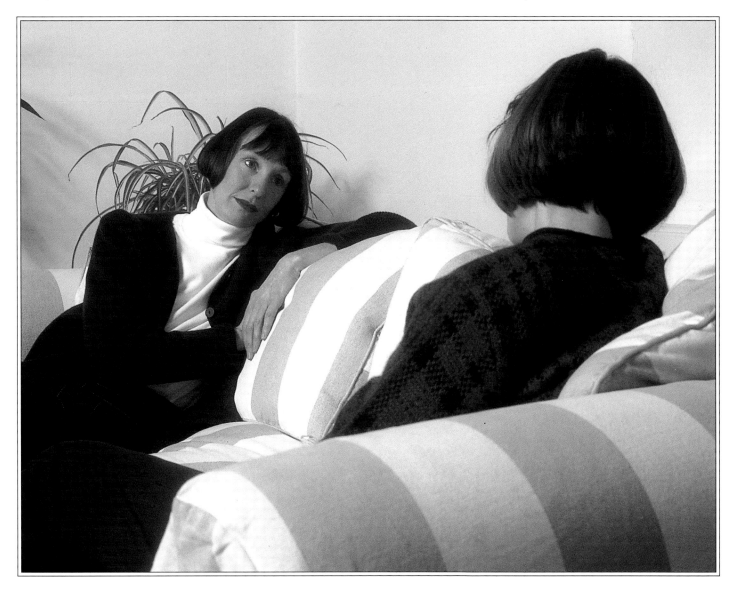

AUTOGENICS

Autogenics is a system of relaxation exercises developed in the late 1920s and 1930s by a German psychiatrist and neurologist, Dr Johannes Schultz. He used hypnotherapy on many of his patients and became aware of the great benefits they gained from the deep state of relaxation brought about under hypnosis. This led him to try to devise a set of exercises to enable people to induce a state of relaxation themselves – the word autogenic means self-originated, or coming from within.

The aim of these exercises is to help switch off the part of the nervous system that produces the "fight or flight" response to stress, and to switch on the relaxation mechanisms. There are essentially six exercises, each focusing on a different sensation, and they may be carried out either lying down or sitting in one of two different ways. No special equipment is required, just the time and space to allow relaxation. The simplicity and effectiveness of autogenics have led to it spreading throughout Europe and America and even to Japan.

Autogenic training is normally carried out by a practitioner with a group of people, with the exercises being learned over several weeks. A feature of the training process can be so-called autogenic discharges, temporary sensations or emotions that can be quite intense and are often followed by a feeling of greater energy. These do not happen to everyone, but are one reason for training with a qualified practitioner, who can explain what they mean.

In a training session these sensations are enhanced and strengthened by the silent repetition of certain phrases, which, when carried out on a regular basis, can have remarkable effects in relieving stress and fatigue symptoms. The release of long-standing stresses can be the reason for the autogenic discharge phenomena.

In a group training situation, an autogenic trainer will probably focus on the first of the above exercises – inducing heaviness and relaxation – for a few weeks so that everyone is confident at performing the exercise. Most autogenic trainers encourage their group members to keep detailed diaries of home practice, and the weekly sessions may begin with a discussion of how everyone has got on in

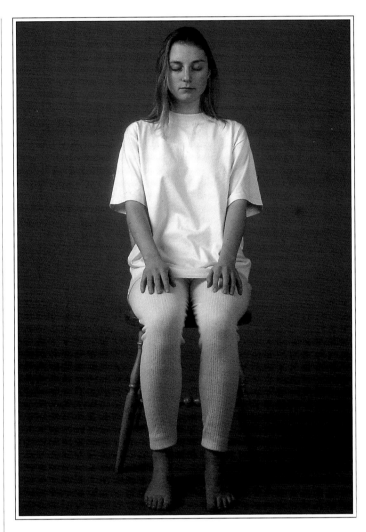

Above: While concentrating on relaxing the body, stress and fatigue are dispelled.

the previous week. This also allows for any individual adjustments that may need to be made to a member's programme.

Initially, repetition of these exercises at home should be just for a couple of minutes, perhaps repeated twice a day; during the course of the sessions, the trainer may well suggest that you increase the length of home exercises to around 15 minutes, two to three times a day. It is important that you fit your exercises into your daily routine so that they become part of your life.

Around 3,000 scientific articles have been published

AUTOGENIC EXERCISE

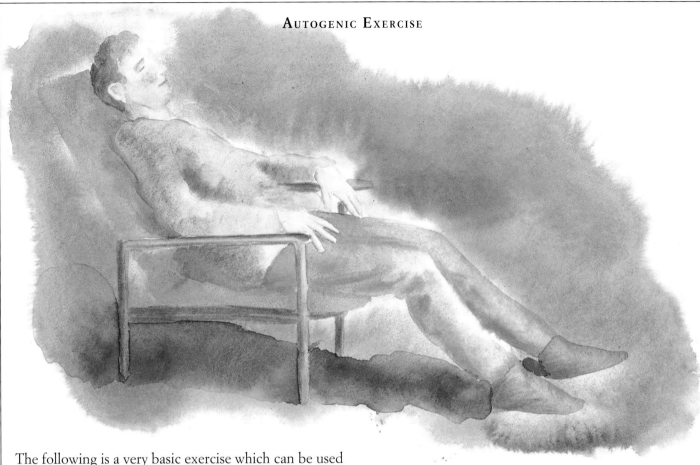

The following is a very basic exercise which can be used as a relaxation technique, using the principles of autogenics to relieve stress:

1 Focus your attention on feelings of heaviness and relaxation in the neck, shoulders and limbs.

2 Develop an awareness of a growing sensation of warmth in the limbs.

3 Concentrate on the heartbeat, and help to regulate it.

4 Build an awareness of your breathing patterns.

5 Create a feeling of warmth in your abdomen.

6 Create a sensation of coolness across the forehead.

describing the beneficial effects of autogenics, although no one can say for certain how the therapy works. Stress-related disorders such as stomach ulcers, migraine, asthma and so on can be improved by these simple exercises. Autogenics are a good example of how mental, emotional and physical health are inextricably intertwined. Repressed emotions or stresses may be responsible for later physical disorders, and this training can help to break this pattern and release the trapped feelings.

The above training exercise can be practised in various places and situations, such as at work, on the train or sitting in a park in your lunch hour. It needs no special clothing or adoption of difficult and awkward positions, and is sometimes compared to learning to drive. First, make yourself comfortable behind the wheel; start off calmly and slowly without any jerks or jolts; next change gear – or alter your

physical and mental states – and finally come to a smooth, safe halt. The exercises above are designed to relieve stress and help the body cure itself. For further exploration into autogenics you should consult a practitioner who will give you a brief check-up to make sure the training is suitable for you. Some patients will only be treated under appropriate medical supervision and modified treatment is given to asthmatics, diabetics, pregnant women and epileptics. Therapists claim that autogenic training can help with a variety of ailments such as AIDS, irritable bowel syndrome, depression and eczema. Many practitioners of autogenics are professionals already involved in healthcare, such as doctors, psychotherapists and psychologists. This probably reflects the depth of research into autogenic training, and has meant that apart from private autogenic practitioners, autogenics may be available through hospitals or general physicians.

HEALING

Healing is based upon the concept that there is more to life than the purely physical; what that something more is depends on your religious or philosophical beliefs. A term that is commonly used is the spirit, although energy is another frequently used expression. For many healers this energy flows from God, or gods in other religions, but nearly all healers agree that this non-physical quality pervades the universe, and is the source of life. Healers claim to have an ability to channel this energy and help it stimulate our own self-healing energies.

For thousands of years healers have practised a number of non-physical methods of focusing attention and healing energy upon people. The most popular method is by the laying on of hands, either directly on to a diseased or affected area of the body or generally over the person receiving heal-

ing. Since there is often a religious element in the beliefs of the healer, or the society in which healers practise, the laying on of hands has often been restricted. In many states in the US, healing is still technically illegal unless you are a church minister, which has led to many people becoming ministers of unusual churches in order to practise. In the UK, it is only within the last 20 years or so that doctors have been able to co-operate with healers without the risk of being struck off the medical register.

There have, nevertheless, been several instances when the benefits of the laying on of hands were recognized within conventional medicine. For example, the former professor

BELOW: The image of healing hands is a powerful one and appears in religions around the world as a symbol of love and care.

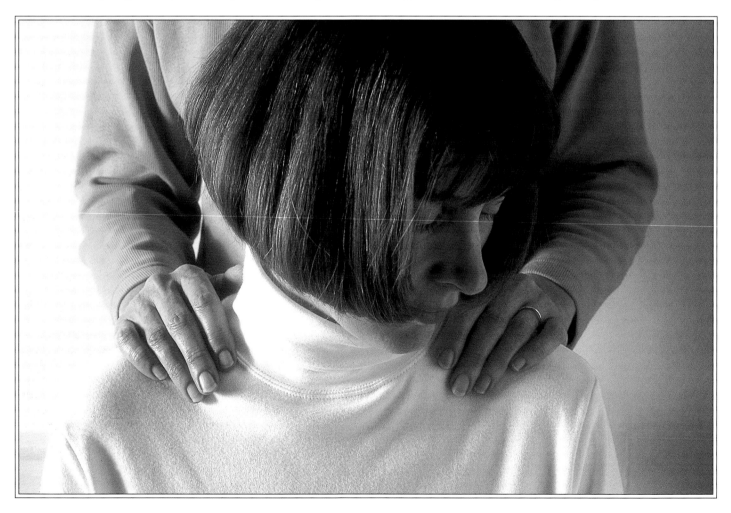

of nursing at New York University, Dr Dolores Krieger, ran a course in "therapeutic touch" (essentially healing by another name) as part of the nurses' training. This proved popular with nurses and patients, and showed not only psychological and emotional benefits for the patients, but quantifiable improvements in health.

In the l980s two lecturers in physiology, Dr David Hodges and Dr Tony Scofield, of London University, conducted controlled experiments to test the curative powers of a psychic healer and medium. This healer claimed he could take cress seeds whose ability to grow had been diminished by a soaking in salt water, and make them well again. The healer held half of the seeds in his hand and directed his healing energy at them. The treated and untreated seeds were then laid on wet tissue paper and left in the lab for a week.

The results were that the "healed" seeds grew significantly faster than the unhealed seeds, leading Dr Hodges and Dr Scofield to conclude that a healing power had enabled the sick seeds to throw off ill-effects and grow normally. This experiment went some way to contradict some medical experts who dismiss the work of healers with the theory of "spontaneous remission" in which the body temporarily heals itself, or auto-suggestion, whereby patients heal themselves by self-hypnosis.

Some healers operate directly within a religious context, giving "faith healing", often in mass gatherings. While healers would acknowledge that faith, either in the healer or in the process, is an important element, it is not generally regarded as essential. Indeed, it is also important that you retain your common sense when seeking a healer. In the last 20 years or so a fair amount of research has started to

Below: Healing is now becoming a more accepted part of modern medicine, with some general practices employing a healer.

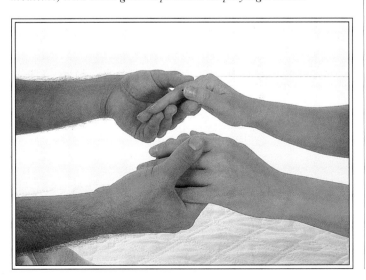

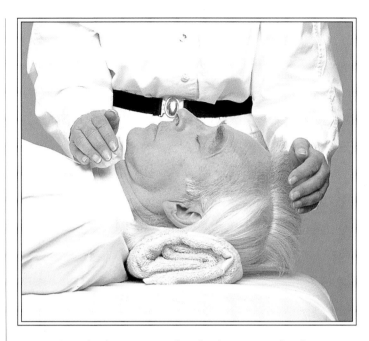

Above: Some healers transmit their healing powers by placing their hands on the patient's aura rather than directly on the body.

accumulate, showing that healers have some ability to affect physical processes by immaterial means. For example, the healer Matthew Manner has carried out many controlled experiments in both the US and the UK with interesting results on cancer cells, and work at the Universities of New York, Wisconsin and Minnesota indicate the benefits of "therapeutic touch". Nevertheless, healing is less amenable to scrutiny than some other therapies, and the possibilities for fraud, or at least misrepresentation, are thus greater.

Despite occasional sensationalized media reports of instant "miracle cures", most healers would say that healing is generally a gradual, slow process. Although, as mentioned above, healers do not as a rule emphasize the need for any faith on the part of the person receiving healing, they would encourage self-healing attempts and above all a positive attitude – the desire to get better. This encouragement of self-help empowerment is a useful guideline to bear in mind when seeing a healer for the first time; if the healer insists on sole responsibility for helping you, to the exclusion of all other treatments, then you are well-advised to look elsewhere.

Most good practitioners of natural medicine probably have some healing abilities, which may be especially evident if they practise a hands-on therapy – for example, massage. Healers concentrate on focusing this healing energy, sometimes with amazing results. Even where there is little or no change in their physical symptoms or illness, many people report that they feel stronger, calmer and more able to cope with their illness after a healing session.

BODYWORK

What is the special importance of bodywork? Simply, it provides the most immediate way to affect another person, to reassure and relax them, to help to reduce pain, influence our ability to build relationships, and even fight off disease. Touch is an absolutely primal, vital requirement that is sadly neglected in many of our

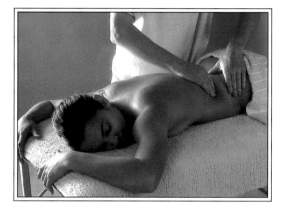

societies. The continuing rise in the popularity of bodywork therapies shows how much this need is still there.

In the last 30 years researchers have started to look at the therapeutic effects of touch, and have shown that not only does regular physical contact lower anxiety levels and enhance the quality of life, but it affects physiological processes, too, ranging from lowered blood pressure, and even less arteriosclerosis, to reduced brain cell deterioration and memory loss with ageing. Musculoskeletal disorders are most often helped by manipulative or other physical treatments, and both pain levels and pain tolerance can often be aided with the help of bodywork therapies.

As if that were not enough, many therapies such as massage are also very enjoyable treatments to receive, and some techniques can be adapted for use at home, helping the giver too. A famous study in the 1960s looked at frequency of touch by couples in cafés around the world; in South America it was 180 times an hour, in the US twice an hour and in England never, so there is much room for improvement.

ABOVE: Professional massage is widely available at natural health centres.

OPPOSITE: Self-massage is often unconscious and with some practice can become part of our daily routine.

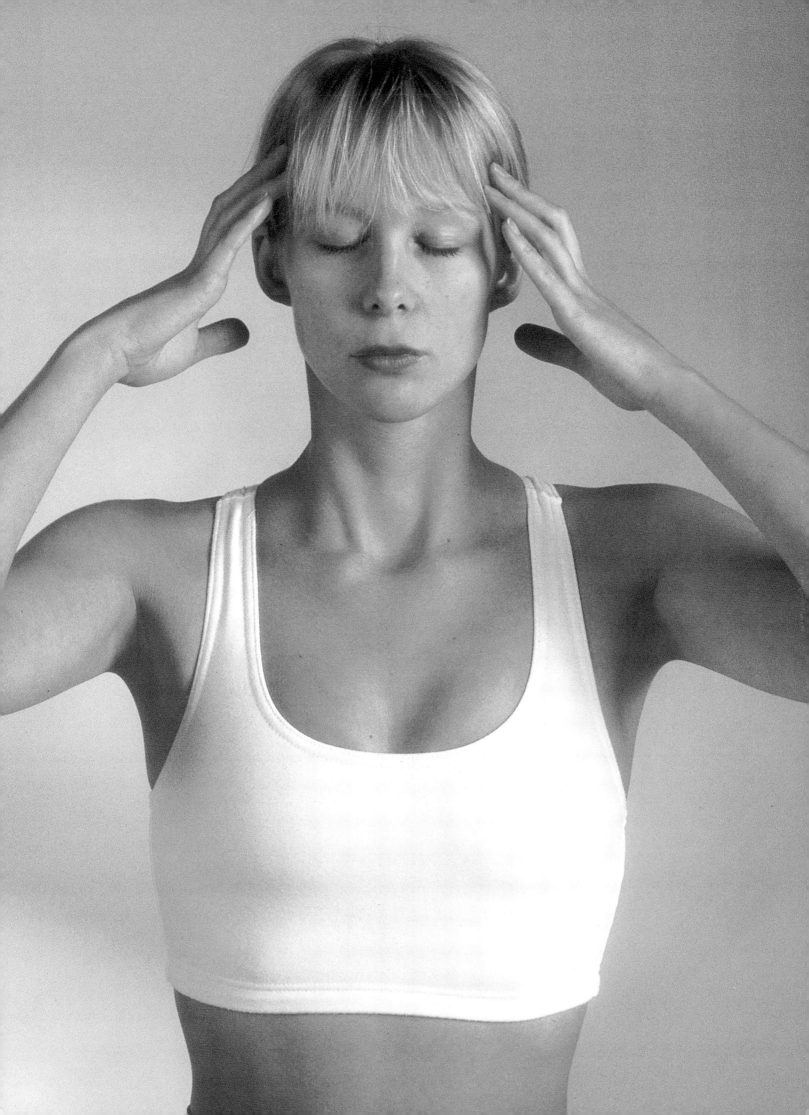

MASSAGE

ORIGINS AND DEVELOPMENT

Massage can fairly claim to be the oldest form of healing in existence. The use of touch to relieve aching muscles, to give comfort or to express love is as old as humankind, and is something humans share with animals as an instinctive way of bonding and sharing. As a stress-reliever it is probably without equal, and every culture throughout history has used massage in some form or other (every language, ancient or modern, has a word for massage).

Written records mentioning massage, or rubbing as it was known in former times, date back some 5,000 years, with the most ancient Chinese medical texts advocating stroking the limbs to "protect against colds, keep the organs supple and prevent minor ailments". In India, the Ayurvedic scriptures, which date back nearly 4,000 years, also recommend rubbing and shampooing the body to keep it healthy and promote healing, and there has been an unbroken tradition of using massage since that time; most Indian mothers are taught to massage their newborn babies, and later the children are taught to massage their parents.

BELOW: Before you begin a massage session prepare some clean, warm towels, some cushions and the oils you will use.

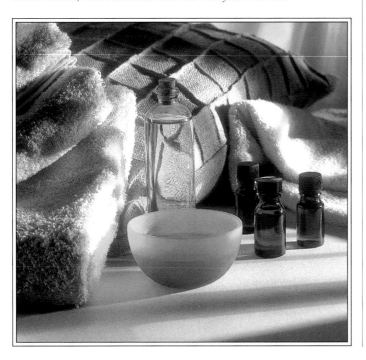

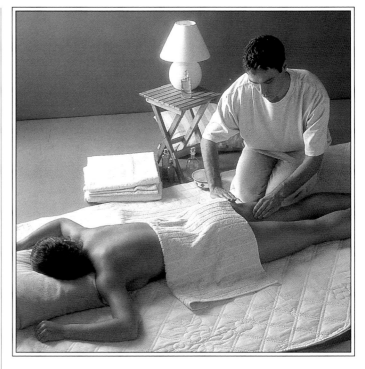

ABOVE: One of the best ways to relax with a partner is to give each other a soothing massage at the end of a stressful day.

In ancient Greece, the practice of rubbing up the limbs, or anatripsis, was highly recommended for treating fatigue, sports or war injury and illness. Hippocrates, the so-called "father" of medicine, writing in the fifth century BC, stated that the physician must be "experienced in many things but assuredly rubbing", and suggested that the way to health was to have a scented bath and an oiled massage each day. Medical centres, or gymnasia, nearly always included massage schools within them.

The Romans were equally enthusiastic about the benefits of massage, incorporating it into a daily routine in their spas, alongside hot and cold baths. One of the most famous Roman physicians, Galen, wrote several books on massage, exercise and health in the second century AD, and classified many types of strokes for use in different ailments. A good masseur was highly regarded.

Massage continued to be popular and respected in Europe after the Romans had left, although their elaborate bathing and massage facilities fell into disrepair. With the rise in more puritanical aspects of Christianity, however, the needs of the body were felt to be in some way sinful and massage became rather neglected.

From the time of the Renaissance, when classical medicine and philosophy were once again in favour, massage was revived and respected again; the French doctor Ambroise Paré, who was physician to no fewer than four French kings, used massage a great deal in his practice. Other cultures had always continued to value massage – Captain Cook wrote in his diaries how he was cured of sciatic pains in Tahiti by being massaged from head to foot by several women at once.

The most influential figure in renewing interest in massage during the nineteenth century was the Swedish gymnast, Per Henrik Ling (1776–1839). Ling studied the human body

in activity and rest, and laid the foundations for modern gymnastics. He developed a system of medical gymnastics, exercises for the joints, and massage, based upon ancient techniques, which led to a Crown appointment and the formation of an institute of massage. His classification of strokes and their effects forms the basis of most Western massage today, and brisker styles of massage are often called Swedish massage.

The latest development of massage happened during the 1960s and 1970s, especially in the US, where personal growth centres – most notably the Esalen Institute – adapted massage into a holistic approach that looked at releasing trapped emotional issues and creating overall health and balance rather than simply easing tired muscles or aching limbs. The American massage therapist George Downing was an early writer on this holistic view of massage, and many schools now teach the subject within this framework.

BELOW: Massaging your partner builds up trust and a feeling of ease, as you show your care for each other using touch.

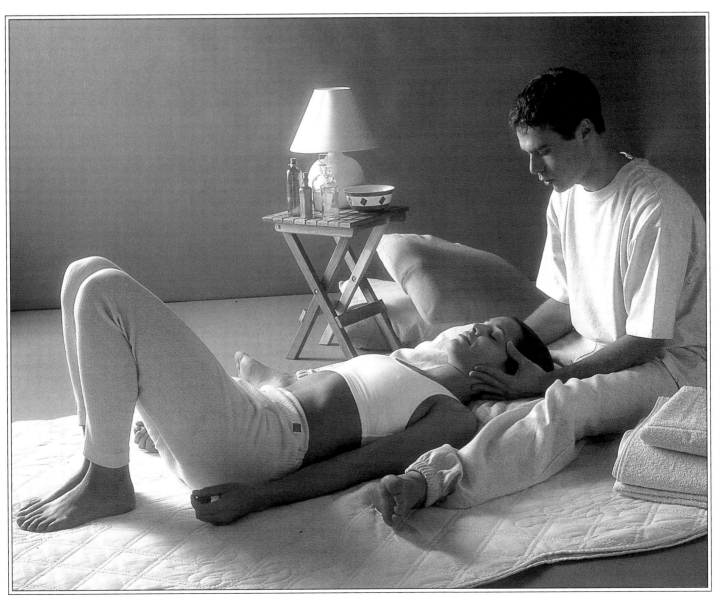

PREVENTIVE MASSAGE

One of the most positive aspects of massage is that you do not need to wait until you have an ailment or injury to receive massage; it is a pleasurable and therapeutic treatment at any time (with few contra-indications), and regular massage is one of the best ways to avoid stress-related illnesses or injury from high levels of exercise and sport. Massage is not appropriate to use where there is an acute infection, feverish condition or inflammation, and care needs to be taken with anyone with heart conditions, so the first rule should be: if in doubt, don't. The suggested strokes outlined below are generally safe, but are not a substitute for professional treatment if needed. They are intended for use in preventing ill-health, not in treating it, and as a means of reducing stress and tension, for yourself and for others.

SELF-MASSAGE

Although often thought of as something you need two people for, massage on yourself is also beneficial and can be done in odd moments during the day. In fact, without perhaps consciously realizing it, every time you rub a tense spot on your shoulder or ease a tight muscle on your forehead you are giving yourself a mini-massage. Use the following techniques throughout the day and you will feel less tired and tense at the end of it.

SHOULDERS AND FACE

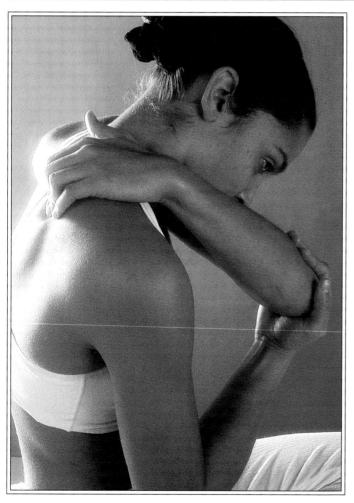

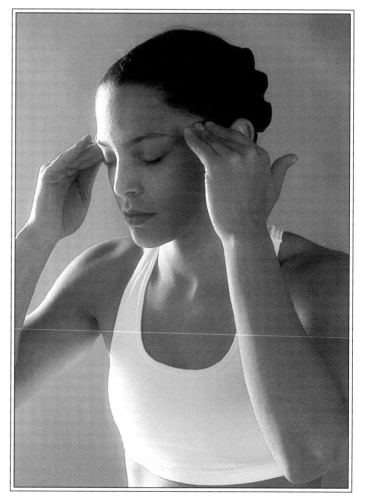

1 A lot of tension can build up in the areas of the shoulders and neck. A regular massage is very helpful, not only giving physical benefits but also breaking up the day and allowing your mind to rest. Squeeze and knead one shoulder firmly with the opposite hand, then change sides and repeat.

2 Try using your fingertips in small, slow circles all over your face, starting at the chin and steadily working upwards. If your shoulders ache from lifting your arms, just pause and rest before starting again, or do this stroke lying on your back on the floor.

HAND MASSAGE

Our hands are one of the most overworked parts of our bodies and will benefit enormously from self-massage throughout the day. People who work with their hands in a repetitive way such as keyboard operators should practise regular hand massage. Hands are also, of course, a vital massage tool and need to be taken care of. Swap hands with each massage technique as you do the following routine.

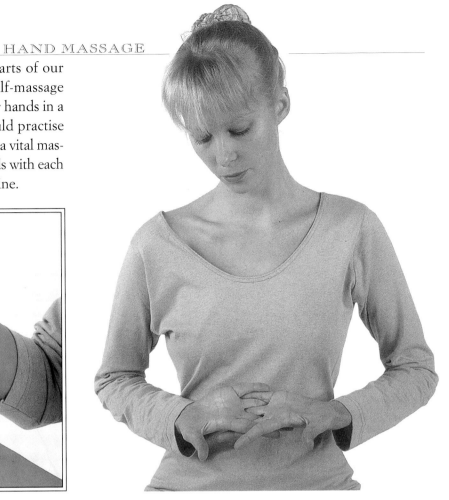

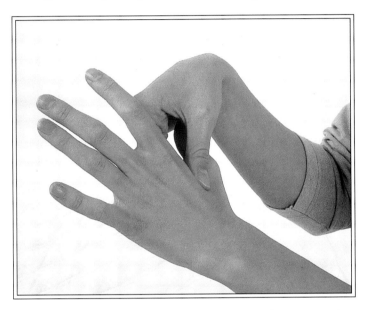

1 To release stored tensions and improve circulation, start by squeezing between each finger in turn with the thumb and index finger of the other hand.

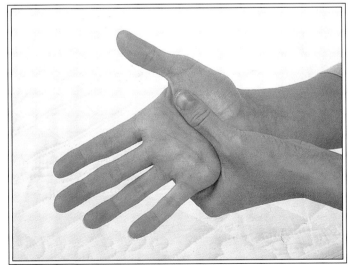

2 Stretch the fingers by interlocking them and gently pulling them downwards. It is not the intention to "crack" the fingers but to stretch the tendons.

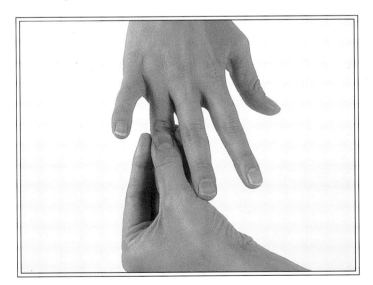

3 Make a rolling movement on each finger, working from the knuckle to the fingertip with firm pressure from the fingers and thumb of each hand.

4 Finally, with the thumb, make a firm circling motion on the palm of the other hand. This both squeezes and stretches taut, contracted muscles and should be a fairly deep action: if done too lightly, it just feels ticklish.

Even when we are not using our arms in a particularly physical way, tiredness induces aching limbs so that we feel physically drained. Use this quick self-massage routine to renew your energy levels during a busy day and prevent any build up of aches and pains.

1 Do a kneading action on the arms, working rapidly from the wrist to the shoulder and back with a firm, squeezing movement. Do this more quickly and briskly than usual in massage, to invigorate each arm and shoulder in turn, rather than soothe and relax the muscles.

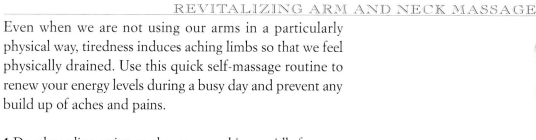

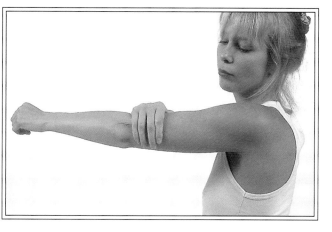

2 Swiftly rub up the outside of each arm using small movements to really stimulate the circulation. Repeat in an upwards direction each time.

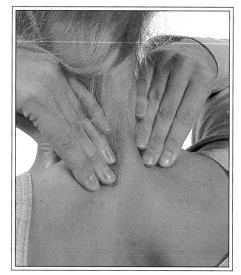

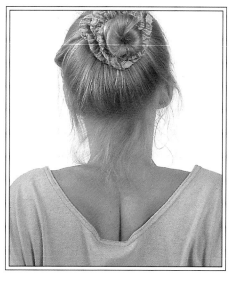

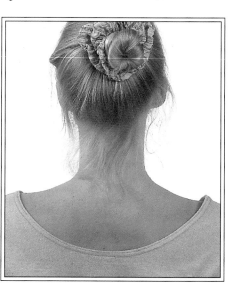

3 With the fingers and thumb of one hand, firmly squeeze the neck muscles with a circular motion.

4 Shrug your shoulders and bring them up close to your ears, hold the position for a few seconds.

5 Relax the shoulders down and feel the tension ebb away. Repeat the exercise two more times.

LEG MASSAGE

This massage is as beneficial to those of us with a sedentary average day as it is for the more physically active. Many of us spend far too long each day standing still, or barely moving around, leading to tired, aching limbs, swollen ankles or cramp. A quick leg massage at the end of the day can work wonders in reducing aches and sluggish blood flow. You could also use this routine in the morning to ease any stiffness. Start on the thighs, so that any fluid retention in the calves will have somewhere to go as the upper leg relaxes.

1 Using both hands, knead one thigh at a time, by squeezing between the fingers and thumb; squeeze with each hand alternately for the best effect. Repeat on the other thigh.

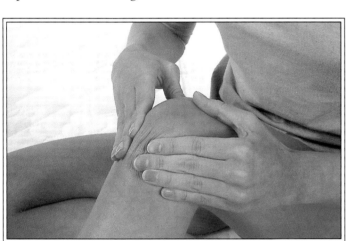

2 Do a similar action around both the knees, but using just the fingers for a lighter effect and working in smaller circles, again squeeze with each hand alternately.

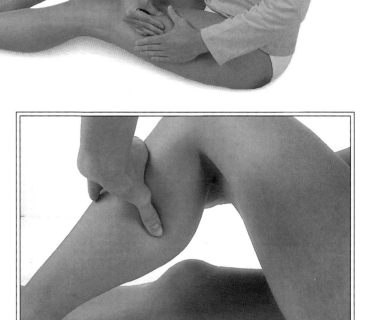

3 Bend the leg and with your thumbs, work up the back of the calf with a circular kneading action. Repeat a few times, each time working from the ankle up the leg.

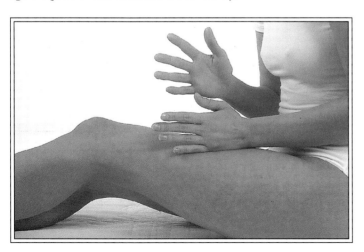

4 With the outside of the hands, lightly hack on the front of each thigh, using a very rapid, almost flicking motion. Keep this action gentle.

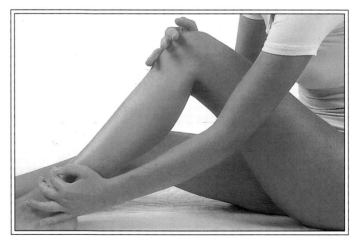

5 Stroke the length of your leg with the fingertips of both hands, from the ankle to the thigh to help blood flow back towards the heart.

MASSAGE WITH A PARTNER

Massaging your partner can be a wonderful way of sharing and giving, helping the relationship as well as easing tensions and preventing stress problems. Preparation is important in order to help release tired, aching muscles and create an overall experience. If you are massaging someone on the floor, use a mattress, quilt or cushions to make a comfortable surface. Cover with a sheet or towels to prevent oil staining your furnishings. Make sure that the room is warm and preferably with softer lighting to help your partner relax.

Aromatic essential oils can be used, but do use a good vegetable oil, such as sweet almond, and avoid thick, sticky mineral oils. The movements suggested below cover the major areas of muscle tension – use as many of them as you need. At the end of the massage, make sure your partner is comfortably wrapped in warm towels and given time to relax and enjoy the full benefit of the massage. Daily massage may not be practical for most people today, but even an occasional one has excellent health benefits.

When giving massage, remember to keep yourself feeling comfortable; breathe freely, try to keep a good posture and let your hands stay as relaxed as possible. If you need extra pressure in any movement, lean in with your whole body and use some of its weight, rather than tensing your fingers. Giving massage can be therapeutic too, and often leaves the giver refreshed and hungry! Above all, enjoy massage, and if in doubt get professional treatment.

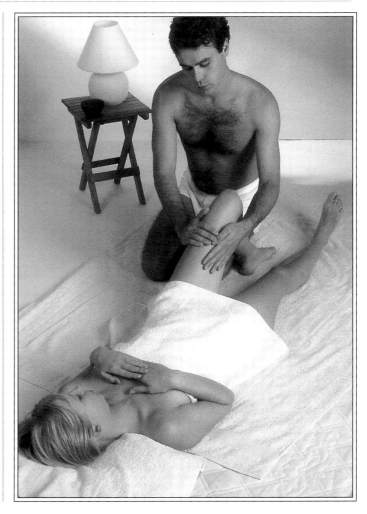

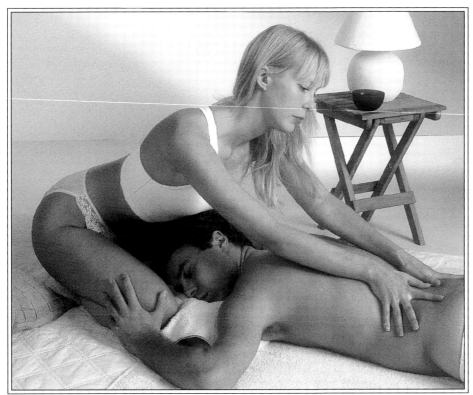

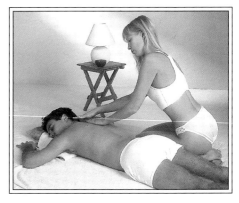

ABOVE AND LEFT: Ensure that your partner is comfortable with what you are doing and the pressure you are using is at the right level – by keeping in touch.

BACK MASSAGE

One of the most reliable ways to relax and unwind – you may find the person being massaged drifts off to sleep – a back massage releases much of the tension we accumulate through the day. Make sure there are no draughts in the room and that your partner is warm and comfortable before you begin. Your oils should be ready and close to hand before you begin so that you don't have to interrupt after you have begun the session. Remember to warm your hands first.

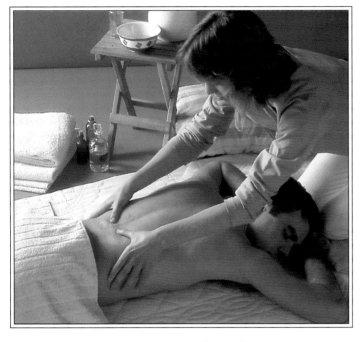

1 Starting on the back, use a smooth, stroking movement downwards with the thumbs on either side of the spine (not pressing on the bones, just outside them) and then take the hands to the side and glide back up the shoulders. Repeat several times.

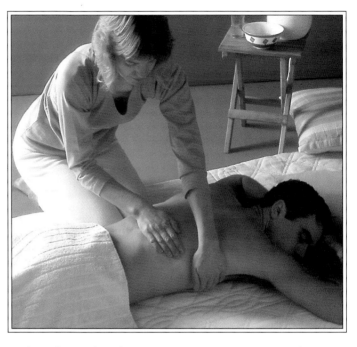

2 Then, from a kneeling position at your partner's side, use the whole of your hands and a smooth stroking movement to pull up steadily, one hand at a time, working all the way up and down one side of your partner's back a few times. Repeat from the other side.

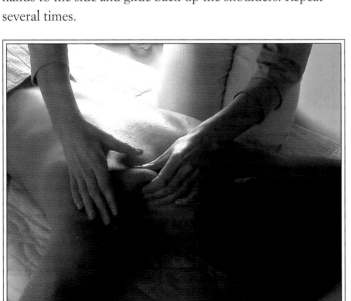

3 Squeeze the muscles from one hand to the other, to knead the muscles of the back and shoulder and release deep-seated muscle tension. Make sure you knead generously rather than using a pinching movement. Repeat on the other side.

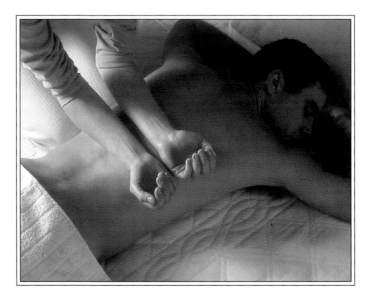

4 Stretch the back, using your forearms to glide in opposite directions. Try to keep a constant, steady pressure, lift off the arms when they reach the neck and buttocks, return to the centre of the back and repeat a few times.

LEGS

This is the perfect massage for the end of a day spent on your feet. It will release those tired aches and pains and leave you feeling relaxed. Do not use any pressure with these movements over varicose veins; if you do anything, just stroke over them lightly towards the heart.

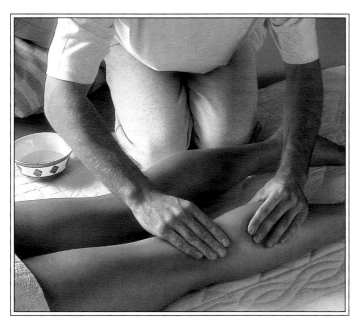

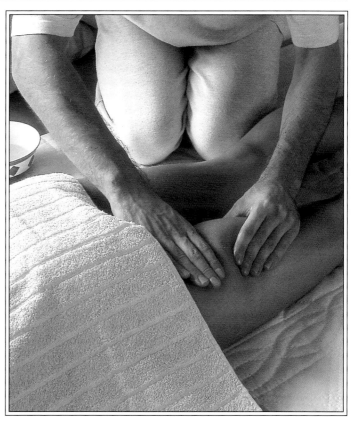

1 Moving down to the back of the legs, knead and squeeze the calf muscles.

2 Do not put any pressure on the area behind the knee, but glide over this and knead the back of the thigh.

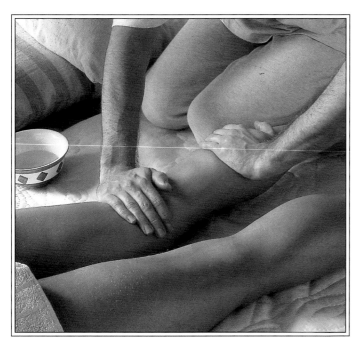

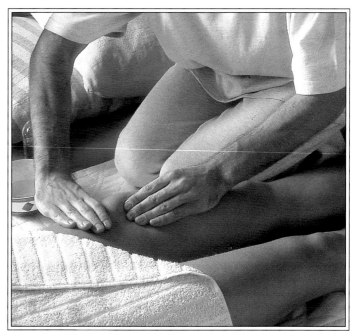

3 Then stroke all the way up the leg, hand over hand, to improve lymph and venous blood flow. Repeat these movements several times, always moving in an upwards direction. Repeat on the other leg.

4 On the front of the legs, kneading of the front of the thighs is helpful, but the front of the lower leg should be avoided as the shin bone is too prominent for this movement. Stroke all the way up the front of the leg and thigh, much as on the back of the leg. Repeat these movements on the other leg.

ABDOMEN MASSAGE

This should be a very gentle action, using a stroking movement and not applying any pressure. Don't do this straight after a heavy meal.

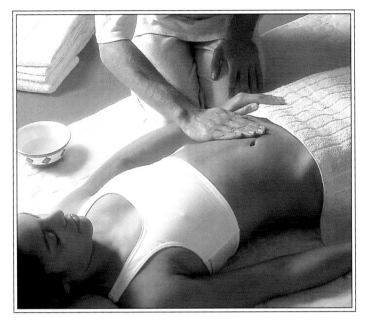

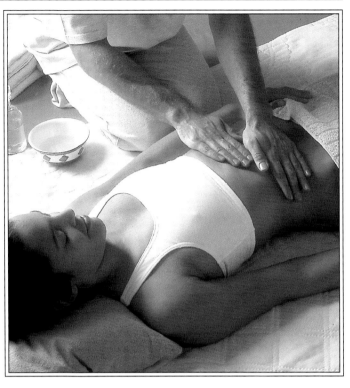

1 On the abdomen, use very slow circling movements in a clockwise direction to aid the digestive process. Make sure your partner is comfortable and relaxed with this movement.

2 Adjust the depth of pressure to your partner's comfort; if done slowly, deeper pressure can be very relaxing but do not overdo it.

ARM AND HAND MASSAGE

When massaging hands remember that some people find light movements ticklish and irritating.

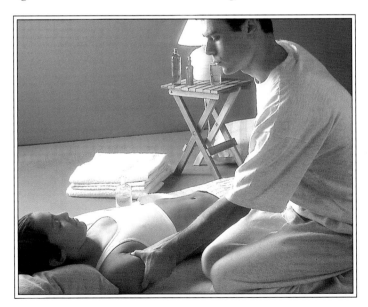

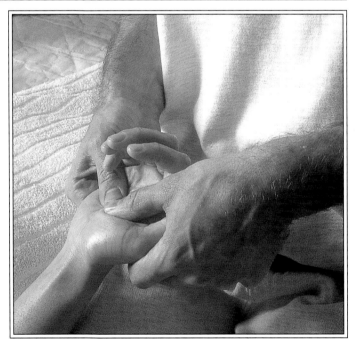

1 For the arms, stroke and gently squeeze down the arm, from the wrist to the armpit, while supporting the arm with your other hand. You may need to swap hands in order to work all round the arm.

2 Then, with your thumbs, firmly massage into the palm of your partner's hand, using small circles. Repeat these movements on the other arm and hand. Use firm pressure to avoid tickling and irritating movements.

FACE

A good head massage can leave the recipient looking quite different as the facial muscles relax and worry lines disappear – you may be able to make your partner look ten years younger in just a few minutes. To massage the face, sit on the floor with your legs open. The person being massaged should lie on their back with their head between your legs. You might like to sit on a cushion. If this position is difficult for you to maintain, sit against a wall or a chair. Ensure you are comfortable before you start, as the benefits of the massage will be lost if you have to move after you have begun.

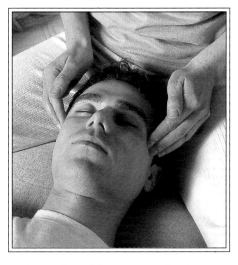

1 The neck and face can be slowly massaged with small circles, using the fingers of both hands working symmetrically to cover all the tiny facial muscles.

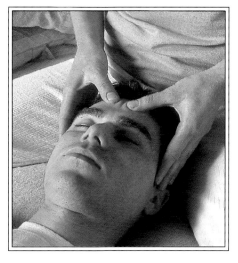

2 Place the thumbs side-by-side on the centre of the forehead and stroke out to the temples, working in strips – smooth away any worry lines.

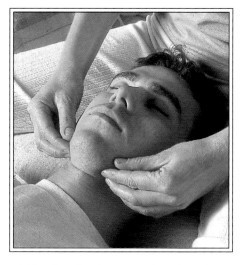

3 Take the chin between thumb and fingers and gently pinch your way out along the jaw, relaxing and releasing any tension.

FINISH

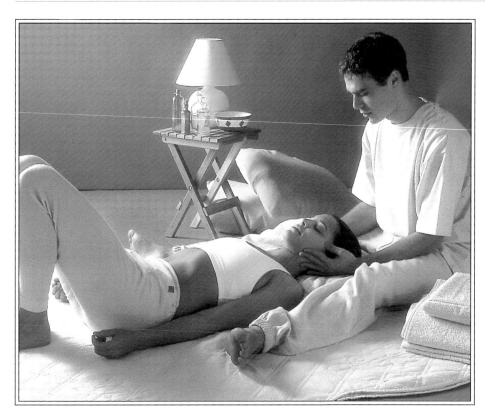

LEFT: If you have worked through all these areas, or even if you choose just one – for example, the back – come to a finish slowly and just place your hands on your partner for a couple of minutes to complete the massage before leaving him or her to rest.

MASSAGE TIPS

If you become tired or short of breath while you are massaging, rest and wait until you have recovered, maintaining contact by keeping one hand on your partner.

Don't wear tight fitting clothes or jewellery while you are massaging.

Make sure that your partner wraps up warmly after you have finished. Have a warmed dressing-gown or bathrobe ready for them to put on.

ROLFING

Rolfing is a system of working on the connective tissues of the body in order to correct imbalances in body posture and restore true alignment. It was founded and developed over some 40 years by Ida Rolf, an American biochemist who died in 1979 aged 84. She was familiar with yoga, osteopathy and other disciplines that might affect the body and health, but felt none of them adequately addressed the problem of restoring vitality and balance. She considered that it was necessary to ensure that the body was working in harmony with the force of gravity, and developed a technique which she originally termed "structural reintegration" to restore this harmony.

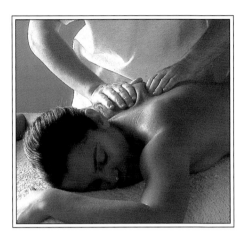

ABOVE: Rolfing can appear to be quite rough, as the connective tissue is manipulated through deep massage.

Ida Rolf gradually created a deep tissue form of massage, to work not so much on the muscles but on the connective tissues that surround muscles, bones and organs. This connective tissue can cover muscles like an envelope, when it is called fascia, or become thickened and bind muscles to bone, or a tendon. If it thickens and binds bone to bone, it is termed a ligament. As rolfers might say, if it fails to do any of these jobs, we call it a pain.

A common reaction of people to rolfing is that it hurts. The techniques can be rather painful at the time, as the practitioner seeks to remould the connective tissue to allow the body to come back into balance with the forces of gravity. Such pain should be only very temporary, however, and can be completely outweighed by the relief of chronic pain and discomfort from poor postural alignment after one or two rolfing sessions. As a general rule, rolfers work through the whole body in about ten sessions, steadily correcting postural faults in different areas through deep manipulative and massage movements.

The first session is essentially a diagnostic one, with the rolfer examining your structure, flexibility and posture, and perhaps taking photographs of how you hold yourself. Polaroids may be taken at the end to show what can be done even in one session. During the following two sessions the legs, shoulders, ribs and pelvis will be worked on to try to bring the body back into alignment with the forces of gravity. In the next sessions the practitioner works on the deeper muscles and tissues of the body, from the inside of the ankles, through thigh and pelvic musculature to the abdomen, back and neck. The final two or three sessions help to link all these areas together.

The whole process is essentially a process of learning about your body, and restoring it so that it can work more efficiently and with less strain. The deep work on the muscles and connective tissues can certainly cause discomfort from long-held tensions and stiffness, but generally this is replaced with a sense of the body becoming strong as the fibres are stretched back to their optimum length.

Since Ida Rolf's death, much of the training work has been carried on by the Rolf Institute in Boulder, Colorado, and practitioners from there have spread out through the US, Europe and beyond. Rolfing's emphasis on working with the connective tissue may indeed make it a painful process, but can have significant health benefits.

BELOW: Rolfing practitioners maintain that deep massage softens the collagen material and remoulds it back into a balanced state.

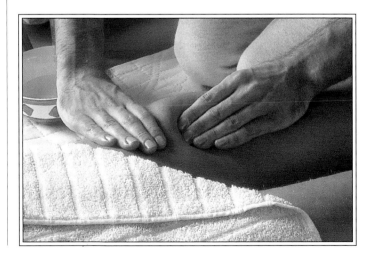

REFLEXOLOGY

The basic concept behind reflexology is that the whole body, indeed the whole person, is interconnected and that imbalances in one part of the body are reflected in changes elsewhere. There are probably some historical connections between the basis for reflexology and other systems, such as acupuncture or acupressure, and writings from ancient Egypt and Rome seem to describe healing points that correspond with reflex zones. It is certainly apparent that both the Incas and the Native Americans used forms of foot massage that are related to reflexology treatments. The latter may have been an influence on Dr William Fitzgerald whose observations and theories laid the foundations of modern reflexology.

Dr Fitzgerald was an American doctor, specializing in the ear, nose and throat area, who practised in the early part of the twentieth century in various hospitals in the US and England. Nobody is quite certain how he arrived at his ideas

BELOW: Reflexology can be practised at home for general relaxation and health but is no substitute for professional treatment which can reduce pain, improve the function of internal organs and also act as a diagnostic tool.

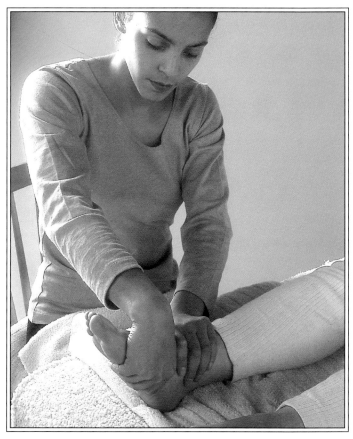

ABOVE: Reflexologists regard the feet as a map of the whole body so that by stimulating a particular point on the foot the therapist balances energy flow and can directly affect an internal organ or gland in the body.

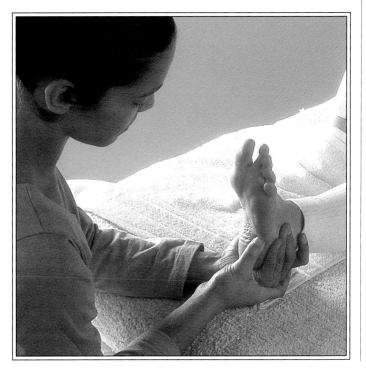

but he discovered that pressure, or massage, on certain parts of the body helped to improve the functioning of internal organs, or else helped to reduce pain sensations. In 1913, he announced his findings, outlining his theory of interconnecting zones within the body – these can be visualized simply as ten vertical strips running the length of the body – with any problems arising in one of these zones being affected by the rest of that zone.

In 1917, Dr Fitzgerald, with his colleague Dr Edwin Bowers, published his ideas and the system of reflex zone therapy was established. It spread among doctors and others in the US, notably a Dr Riley who created a highly successful practice and expanded on the theories behind

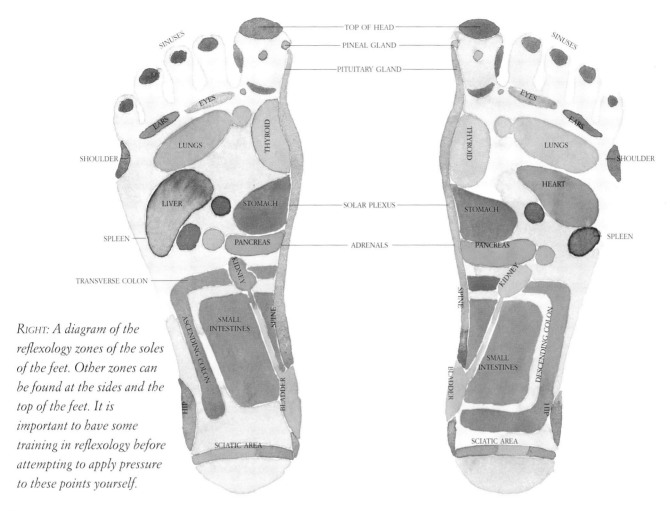

TOP OF HEAD
PINEAL GLAND
PITUITARY GLAND
SINUSES
EYES
EARS
SHOULDER
LUNGS
THYROID
LIVER
STOMACH
SOLAR PLEXUS
SPLEEN
PANCREAS
ADRENALS
KIDNEY
TRANSVERSE COLON
ASCENDING COLON
SMALL INTESTINES
SPINE
HIP
BLADDER
SCIATIC AREA

SINUSES
EYES
EARS
SHOULDER
THYROID
LUNGS
HEART
STOMACH
SPLEEN
PANCREAS
KIDNEY
SPINE
DESCENDING COLON
SMALL INTESTINES
BLADDER
HIP
SCIATIC AREA

RIGHT: A diagram of the reflexology zones of the soles of the feet. Other zones can be found at the sides and the top of the feet. It is important to have some training in reflexology before attempting to apply pressure to these points yourself.

reflexology. Dr Riley taught an assistant, Eunice Ingham, who popularized reflexology through a couple of influential books, *Stories the Feet Can Tell* and *Stories the Feet Have Told*. Unlike Dr Fitzgerald, who worked on various areas within the zones such as the hands, feet, lips, nose and ears, Eunice Ingham concentrated on the feet. She believed that since they contained points relating to all ten zones, they were of special significance in treatment.

Ingham's ideas about what reflexology did were rather simplistic, and are outdated nowadays, but they helped to focus treatment via the feet. She developed the theory that, with slower circulation to the extremities, tiny crystalline deposits occur around various nerve endings in the feet, much as silt forms in a river as the current slows. The reflexologist uses firm pressure to crush these little crystals and restore normal functioning. This theory is just one view of how reflexology works: no one has really come up with a comprehensive explanation and most practitioners today discuss its effects in terms of balancing energy flow (in similar fashion to Oriental systems of medicine).

Reflexology has expanded in popularity greatly across the world in the last 30 years. This is partly due to its relative simplicity as a non-invasive method of treatment, and partly

from the plain fact that although nobody has successfully explained why it should work, it does. There have been some recent studies – for instance, one carried out by nurses at a hospital in Manchester, England – which demonstrated the benefits of reflexology in reducing the symptoms of stress, and increasing numbers of natural therapists are recognizing its value.

Reflexology is of considerable benefit in stress-related ailments, in reducing pain and in improving the functioning of internal organs; it also has some usefulness as a diagnostic aid, as tender reflex points can help to locate areas of dysfunction. Gentle, generalized foot massage techniques are suitable for home use too, to maintain good health, although they are not a substitute for professional treatment.

Stretching and loosening the feet will in itself improve local circulation and help general relaxation. Using steady, fairly firm pressure, you may locate tender spots on the feet. These should be treated with great gentleness and should not be pressed too hard or for too long, as this can produce a strong reaction in the affected area of the body. The thumbs are normally used, although fingers may be more useful in some places. Any tenderness at the end of the massage can be eased by soothing or rubbing the feet afterwards.

FOOT MASSAGE WITH A PARTNER

Arrange for your partner to be warm and comfortable; sitting on a chair with a section for the feet that can be raised, or lying on a bed may be appropriate. Ideally, your partner's feet should be almost up to the level of your shoulders. Make sure that you too are comfortable before beginning so that you do not have to alter your position. Oil can be used for foot massage, but the direct pressure technique does work better without it, so that your hands do not slip.

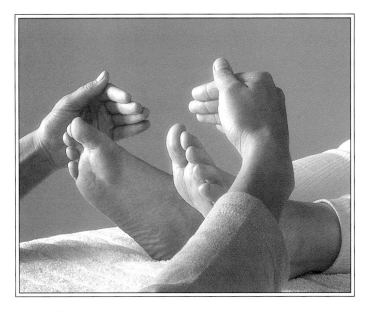

1 Initially, simply make contact with your partner's feet, by curving your hands over the top of them just a few inches away. This is called "greeting the feet" and its steady contact can be very relaxing and reassuring in itself. Our feet carry us around all day, with really very little protest, but tensions do build up in them and stretching movements can help to revitalize us very quickly, without the need of detailed treatment on specific reflexology points.

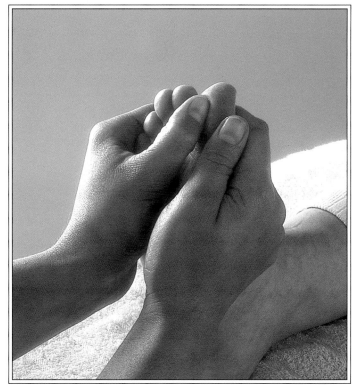

2 Massage each toe in turn using your thumb, then flex and extend them gently. Gently twist the foot sideways to stretch all the muscles.

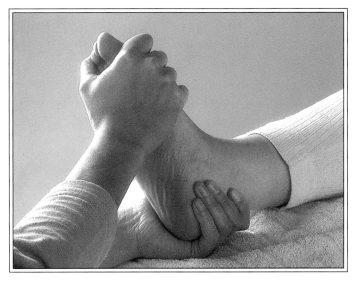

3 Holding the top of the foot with one hand and cupping the heel in your other hand, use the top hand to flex and extend the whole foot, steadily, to loosen up all the joints.

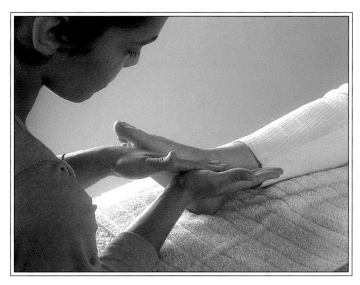

4 If your partner is tired and exhausted, the feet and indeed the whole system can be reinvigorated by hitting the inside edge of the foot lightly with the side of your hands. Only use this movement if someone needs to be woken up.

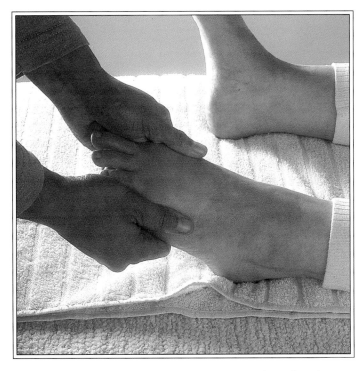

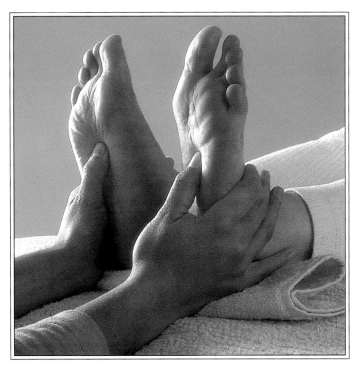

5 Then ease out tensions in the lateral arch of the foot by holding the foot with both hands, one on each side, and stretching across the top of the foot in a movement rather like breaking open a crusty bread roll.

6 A final and very helpful relaxing pressure can be given on the reflex points that relate to the solar plexus. This is often called the brain of the abdomen, and is a huge collection of nerve fibres that controls the digestive organs. The points on the feet are located between the big toe and the next toe, just below the large pad beneath the big toe; pressing both feet at the same time is more effective.

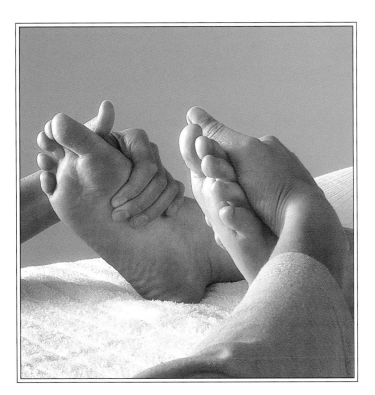

7 To finish hold the feet by resting your hands gently on top of them for a few minutes and slowly breaking contact, helping your partner to unwind completely.

BENEFITS OF REFLEXOLOGY

Reflexology has been used to treat a number of common ailments including back pain, digestive problems, migraine, menstrual problems, sinus problems and general stress and tension. It has also been used for more serious ailments such as heart disorders and multiple sclerosis. It is also thought that a reflexologist can sometimes detect an impending illness and give preventive treatment, if appropriate, or advise the patient to see a specialist. By having regular treatment, perhaps every month or so, good health may be maintained and early warning signs spotted. Reflexology can have quite powerful effects and is therefore better avoided by pregnant women or people with arthritis, osteoporosis or heart and thyroid disorders. As a home therapy, however, reflexology massage should be restricted to a gentle relaxation method. You can try these simple movements on yourself, and if this is difficult the same effects can be produced by massaging the corresponding points on your hand.

CHIROPRACTIC

Chiropractic is a well-established system of treatment and, alongside osteopathy, is respected as one of the major forms of manipulative therapy. It is based upon the premise that structure affects function, and in particular that displacement of the structure of the spine can cause pressure on nerves which in turn affect other parts of the body. In the US it is extremely popular, with around 50,000 chiropractors in practice, and it is also widespread in Australia. In the UK there are currently more osteopaths than chiropractors, but both are accepted by the medical profession.

In 1895, in Iowa, a self-taught "magnetic healer" named Daniel David Palmer treated his office janitor, who had become deaf after bending over and feeling a click in his back. Palmer discovered a slight misalignment of the man's spine and manipulated the bones to restore true alignment; this led to the hearing being restored. Subsequently, Palmer went on to found a school of chiropractic – the word derives from two Greek words meaning practical use of the hand.

Chiropractors use a variety of manual adjustment techniques to help correct faulty alignment, and following a thorough physical examination, plus questioning about your general health, are likely to take X-rays to establish precisely what is happening to your skeleton. Manipulation is then carried out to give normal movement back to any affected joints, and you will probably be re-examined to make sure that the joints are now moving more freely. In chronic or severe cases, a series of treatments may be necessary.

The vast majority of people seeking chiropractic treatment suffer from some kind of musculoskeletal pain, especially in the neck or lower back. A common injury caused by car accidents is whiplash, where the head and neck are abruptly jerked, and chiropractors can often correct the trauma caused to the structures. Frequent headaches may also be a reason for a visit to a chiropractor, and relief is often reported from the manipulative adjustments.

Although some chiropractors restrict themselves completely to spinal adjustments, many practitioners, especially in the US, may give advice on exercise and nutrition, and even prescribe dietary supplements. This is similar to some schools of training in osteopathy which combine advice with naturopathy for all-round health benefits. The manipulative treatments have been the subject of some research, and in American, English and New Zealand studies, for instance, chiropractic has been shown to be one of the most effective forms of treatment for musculoskeletal problems.

The differences between chiropractic and osteopathy are largely historical, and both systems accept modern physiological ideas, mainly differing in the specific techniques used to achieve similar aims. That chiropractic treatment is covered by Medicare, Medicaid and most health insurance schemes in the US, and some in the UK, is a sure sign that the manipulative therapies have established their credentials.

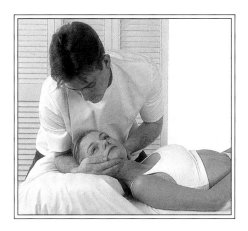

ABOVE: *Chiropractic often involves a sudden movement which results in a "clicking" sound as the bones are realigned.*

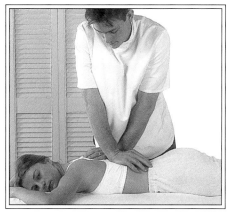

ABOVE: *Backache is often linked to an injury sustained earlier in life and can be easily and effectively cured by chiropractic.*

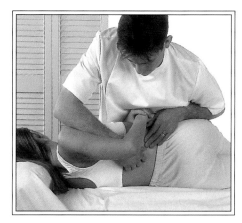

ABOVE: *The practitioner sometimes uses his or her body weight to realign the bones, which can be alarming but is perfectly safe.*

CRANIO-SACRAL THERAPY

Cranio-sacral therapy has grown out of an osteopathic background, and an increasing number of osteopaths are including or even specializing in cranial osteopathic techniques. Cranio-sacral therapy is also taught and practised by other therapists (with some disapproval from osteopathic circles); probably the most fundamental quality needed from a practitioner is great sensitivity of touch.

Its origins date back to an American osteopathic physician, William Garner Sutherland, practising in the early years of the twentieth century. He developed the theory that the skull, which consists of eight bones joined by fine sutures, was able to expand and contract marginally, and did so in response to the rhythmic flow of cerebro-spinal fluid within the brain and spinal column. As this fluid wells up within the ventricles, deep inside the brain, it affects the membranes supporting the brain and in turn increases pressure on the cranium itself.

Dr Sutherland carried out experiments on himself, using various contraptions to stop his skull moving, with many startling results on his physical health and behaviour. This

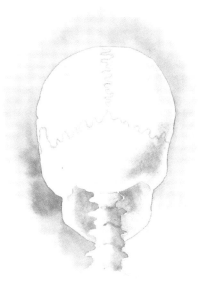

ABOVE: The cranium and its fluids are mobilized in cranio-sacral therapy.

led him to advocate very gentle manipulative movements, to mobilize the cranio-sacral rhythmic flow of fluid and allow this expansion/contraction to occur naturally and without any impediment. He theorized that any blow or trauma, from birth onwards, could impair this system, and lead to ill-health of many kinds.

Sutherland's theories were largely dismissed by orthodox medicine in his time; but modern medical research, notably at Michigan State University, has demonstrated that much of what Sutherland suggested has a good scientific basis.

Cranial techniques can be of particular benefit to young children, and this is an expanding field. One of the first people to work with Sutherland was a pediatrician, Dr Beryl Arbuckle, who became world-famous for her work with cerebral palsy sufferers. What is less known is that her osteopathic approach was almost entirely cranial. The Osteopathic Centre for Children in London also uses cranial work to a large, and successful, extent.

Conditions where cranial techniques may prove valuable include headaches, pains originating in the tempero-mandibular (jaw) joint, and recurrent ear and sinus infections in children. These examples may not seem surprising, but this therapy may also benefit children who have had birth traumas, brain injuries, or developmental and behavioural problems such as hyperactivity. Indeed, children can sometimes respond dramatically quickly to cranial work.

The rather unconventional theories behind cranio-sacral therapy, and the considerable sensitivity required from the practitioner, are probably the main obstacles to it becoming more widespread. The touch of a therapist is very light and yet quite profound changes are reported, and this can be disconcerting for some people. Apart from cranial osteopaths, most people who train in cranio-sacral therapy tend to be bodywork practitioners already, with high levels of palpatory ability as well as professional therapeutic skills, and their numbers are slowly but definitely growing.

BELOW: One of the gentlest therapies, cranio-sacral therapy can alleviate headaches and sinus pain, especially in children.

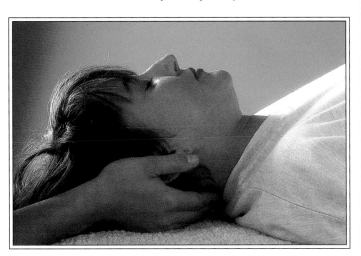

OSTEOPATHY

Osteopathy is one of the two major systems of manipulative therapy, together with chiropractic. Its origins date back to the nineteenth century, but it has philosophical connections right back to the Hippocratic school of medical thought in the fourth century BC. It was founded by an American doctor, Andrew Taylor Still, in 1874, after several years of trying to find a better way of treating his patients than bleeding and purging. He based his ideas on the ancient notion that the body can cure itself, and on the concept of the need for the structure of the body to be correctly aligned in order to release our innate self-healing power.

Although we stand upright our anatomy is still basically that of a creature which moves on all fours, and there is a constant strain on the whole framework. Still recognized that the effect of gravity is particularly severe on the spine, the vertebrae and the cushioning discs between them. Still's earlier training as an engineer helped him in his assessment of the problems that could result from misalignment of the patient's skeletal structure, and his philosophical outlook emphasized the interconnectedness of the body and its self-healing potential.

Still therefore developed the use of manipulative techniques to treat not just the spine but the whole body. Structure and function were seen as interdependent, and attention to the former would improve the latter. In 1892, he founded the first school of osteopathy, in Missouri. One of his students, John Littlejohn, subsequently founded the British School of Osteopathy in 1917. In the US, osteopaths are also medically trained, and represent some five per cent of American doctors; in the UK they considerably outnumber chiropractors, and have recently been granted State Registration as a recognized and statutorily regulated profession.

Osteopathic treatments will involve a detailed case his-

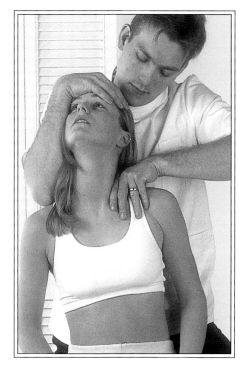

ABOVE: Many hospitals and general practices now employ an osteopath to support conventional treatments.

tory of your general health, as well as particulars of any accidents/injuries and the current problem, and then a complete physical examination to assess the range and freedom of movement of the body. Manipulative techniques, perhaps accompanied by some deep neuro-muscular massage, may be used to help to restore normal structural balance and functioning.

A number of specific techniques have been developed over the last hundred years or so, ranging from gentle, repeated movements of joints to increase their mobility, to quick thrust movements which rapidly guide the joint through its normal range. These latter manipulations can often cause the characteristic clicking noise that many people experience during a session. They may also temporarily irritate surrounding tissues and give some extra discomfort until the area settles down again.

A fairly recent development within some schools of osteopathy has been the use of cranial-osteopathic treatment. This involves very gentle movements to help the flow of cerebro-spinal fluid, a lymph-like fluid which moves rhythmically around the brain and spinal cord, bathing and nourishing the nerve tissues. Any impediment in this rhythm is seen as creating imbalance within the body, with subsequent ill-health (see also *Cranio-sacral Therapy*). Cranial-osteopathic treatments are especially helpful for infants – say, after a difficult birth – and in London, for example, there is an osteopathic hospital centre for children that uses these gentle methods in such circumstances.

Since osteopaths in America may also be family doctors, and in the UK they are not only State Registered but are starting to work in doctors' surgeries or even hospitals, osteopathy has become well integrated into conventional medicine; however, not all doctors accept that it is anything more than just a "back treatment".

ALEXANDER TECHNIQUE

The Alexander Technique is a method of training in posture, body movement and positioning. It was originally devised by Frederick Alexander, an Australian actor, around the turn of the twentieth century. He found that when he was giving an important Shakespearean speech on stage, his voice continually faltered. The only advice given to him was to rest his voice, which only helped until the next large role. Eventually, he set about studying exactly how he was using his body by watching himself in a mirror, and discovered that he tensed his body when performing. The effort of projecting his voice made him bring his head down, restricting his vocal cords and impairing deep breathing or voice control.

Over a period of time Alexander slowly adapted the way he held his body when acting on stage, and overcame this "startle reflex pattern" as he called it. Gradually he developed the idea that body use – how we hold ourselves, move and so forth – can affect the functioning of our internal organs and overall health. He started to teach his methods of body realignment, moving to London in 1904 and subsequently going to the US gaining widespread recognition.

The techniques he devised are based upon the principle of extending the spine, allowing it to reach its optimal length, and generally to redeploy the body's entire muscular system. Exercises are thus geared to restoring natural posture and ease of movement, with minimal muscular effort. A common phrase used to describe the ideal movement is, "the head leads, the spine follows."

Animals and young children usually move naturally, with a lengthened spine and a sense of poise. Unfortunately, we often acquire bad habits as we get older, and additional stresses can lead to imbalanced and excessive muscular effort in movement. If chronic tensions build up, the neck and back muscles contract, leading to rounded shoulders, a lowered head and an arched back, which causes further tension and so the problem gets worse and worse. Alexander teachers seek to help re-educate us to change these patterns and regain positive, easy body use.

Alexander schools have often been associated

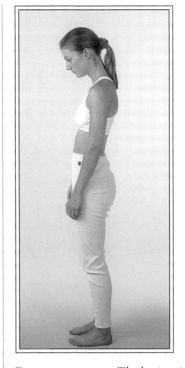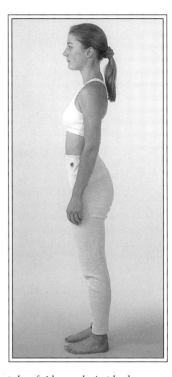

FAR LEFT AND ABOVE: The basic principle of Alexander's ideal posture is to keep your body in a straight line.

with drama or music establishments, echoing the man's background, but the techniques are suitable for all kinds of occupations. Improvements in posture can be accompanied by health benefits such as greater mental alertness, better sleep, increased resistance to stress and enhanced performance of physical tasks. The techniques are learned from a teacher, in the form of lessons rather than treatment sessions, and may initially involve simple actions such as sitting down and getting up from a chair or walking to and fro, with corrective advice on how to use the body more efficiently.

Self-help measures may be of benefit in the first instance; copying Alexander's example and looking closely at your posture in the mirror might be valuable in identifying obvious imbalances. However, since bad habits can be difficult to change, or even spot sometimes, a series of lessons from a teacher is likely to be the most helpful way to correct these.

The Alexander technique is not a cure-all, but improvements in the way we hold and use our bodies can improve many people's overall health and movement.

EASTERN APPROACHES

The traditional Oriental view of health is quite different from the reductionist standpoint of modern, technological medicine in the West. In Eastern philosophy, illness is placed in the context of a holistic approach to life, and in particular the concept of an energy-based system. From the idea of a universal energy, or the highest level of spirituality, down to the lowest forms of life, much of Eastern ideology is an energetic one, with all parts of the human body interconnected and infused with a vital energy, and all life-forms similarly interdependent on an exchange of energies.

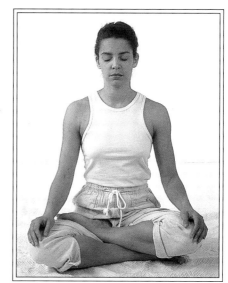

These concepts have led to the development of traditional therapeutic systems, such as acupuncture in China, shiatsu or acupressure in Japan, and yoga in India. Some of these are more suited to professional treatment of ailments, or imbalances in energy flow as they would be described, while practices such as yoga are very suitable for everyday life, in order to *prevent* illness as well as to promote self-development.

Modern medicine in many Far Eastern countries is now often an amalgam of conventional Western medicines alongside traditional approaches; they are quite happy to utilize the best of both worlds, and this is perhaps a useful pointer to the rest of us. Acute, severe illness may be treated with hi-tech medicine, but a more holistic approach can remedy most health problems.

Above: Yoga is one of the most ancient ways of releasing the mind.

Opposite: Acupuncture, once practised only in the East, is now available throughout the world.

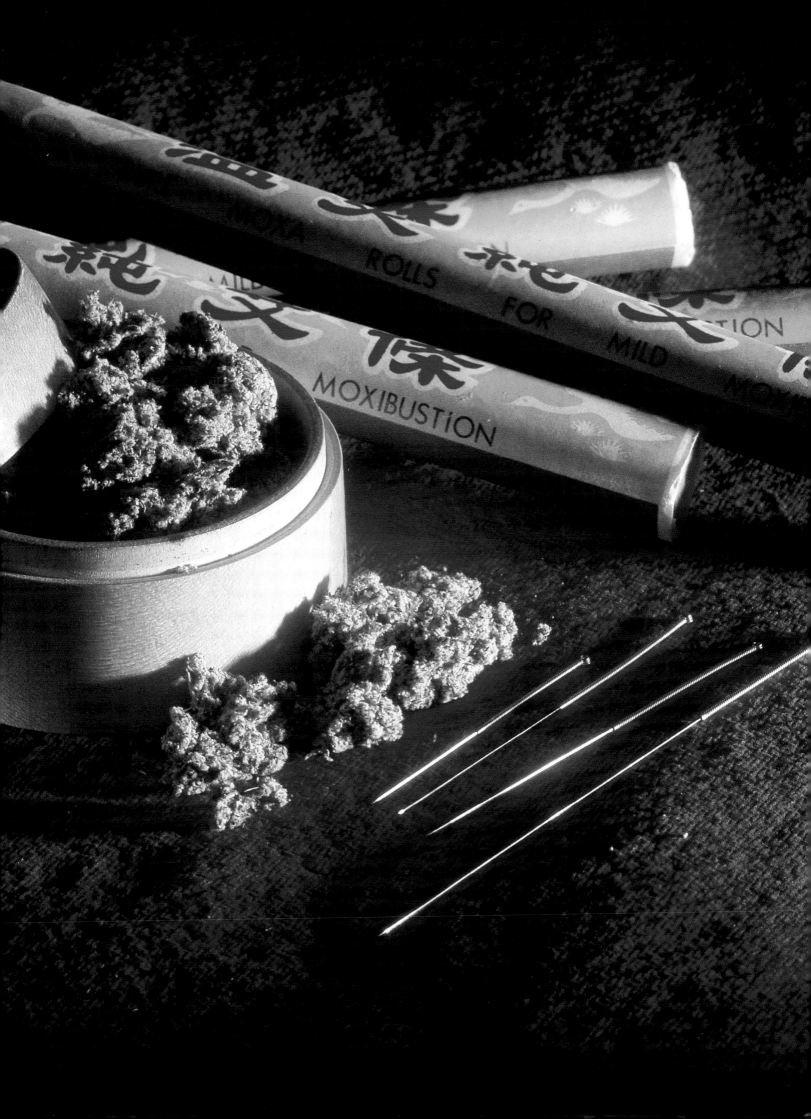

SHIATSU

S hiatsu is a contemporary therapy with its roots in Oriental traditional medicine. It is sometimes described as Japanese physiotherapy since it is primarily a physically based "bodywork" system of treatment. The actual treatment approach and philosophy is similar to acupuncture in its usage of the meridians (energy channels) and *tsubo* (pressure points) as well as diagnostic methods, but without the use of needles. Unlike most other forms of bodywork, in shiatsu the receiver remains clothed for the treatment and this is often a consideration for patients.

The word "shiatsu" is Japanese and literally means "finger pressure". The application of pressure is the underlying principle of shiatsu. This pressure can be applied using not only your fingers, but also the palms of your hands, thumbs, elbows or knees, depending on the amount of stimulation required and which body area is treated. Stretching exercises and other corrective techniques will also be included in the treatment with the intention of creating flexibility and balance in the body, both physically and energetically.

Shiatsu works on the flow of energy or *qi* that circulates through our bodies in specific energy channels or meridians. Essentially, we all have a "life force" or "life energy" which created our physical structure and regulates physical, emotional, mental and spiritual stability. This life force, called *qi* in Chinese and *ki* in Japanese, maintains a homeostatic balance in your body.

The flow of *qi* can be disturbed either through external trauma, such as an injury, or internal trauma such as depression or stress. This is when symptoms like aches and pain start to occur and we start to experience a state of "dis-ease". In shiatsu the physical touch is used to assess the distribution of *qi* throughout the body and to try to correct any imbalances accordingly.

Touch is the essence of shiatsu and a wonderful means of communicating our love and compassion for others in a very direct way. Touch can be of very different quality, ranging from aggressive, abusive and mechanical to more nurturing, caring and intuitive. We all need to be touched in some way and shiatsu helps to fulfil this need. The caring touch used in shiatsu will help to trigger the self-healing process within.

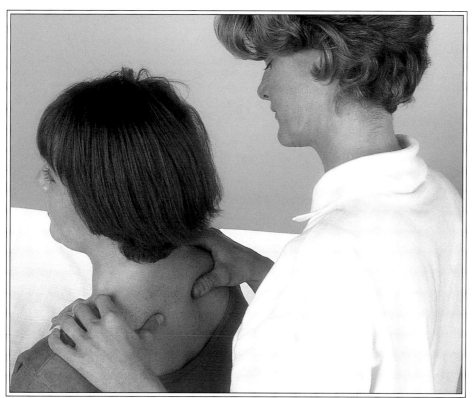

LEFT: The essence of shiatsu is touch. The practitioner will build up a relationship of trust and care with the patient.

SHIATSU AT HOME

The exercises in this chapter give two routines, one which you can do on yourself and one with a partner. You may find that during or at the end of these routines you feel slight mood changes. Other reactions experienced after a professional treatment include cold or mild flu symptoms which disappear after a day or so. Do not attempt any shiatsu techniques other than the following exercises without consulting a trained practitioner.

THE HISTORY AND PHILOSOPHY

Oriental medicine developed out of a need to maintain good health and prevent illness. Therapies such as acupuncture, herbalism, moxibustion (the burning of the mugwort herb on the skin) and *amma* (Chinese massage) developed in different geographical areas according to lifestyle and cultural considerations. In the earliest recorded writing on Chinese medicine, *The Yellow Emperor's Canon of Internal Medicine*, written over 2,000 years ago, the Yellow Emperor asked the master of Oriental medicine why there were so many methods to treat one illness and why each method was effective. The master replied that environment was the main reason for using different approaches. In the east where the people lived close to the sea, tended to eat more fish and protein and suffered skin diseases, acupuncture developed as an effective treatment. In the west, where there are mountains and deserts, the people tended to be fat and eat too much animal protein. This caused problems with their internal organs which were best remedied by herbal medicine. In the cold northern mountainous regions, moxibustion was most effective in driving out respiratory disorders associated with the climate, such as coughing and mucus. In the flat central regions, the people developed symptoms of general weakness which was most effectively treated with *amma* and corrective exercises.

Amma (*anma* in Japanese) has been used for centuries to deal with many common ailments, aches and pains as well as treating more serious "dis-eases". New influences from traditional Eastern medicine and Western science have gradually shaped it into what is today called shiatsu. There are several main styles of shiatsu found in the West: barefoot shiatsu, macrobiotic shiatsu, Namikoshi style, Ohashiatsu, Shiatsu-Do and Zen shiatsu. These are all valid and effective therapies using the basic shiatsu principles but with differing emphasis placed on techniques or philosophy. In Japan there are more than 87,000 registered shiatsu practitioners. This fact alone goes some way towards demonstrating its effectiveness in the prevention and treatment of disease.

QI – YOUR LIFE FORCE

Shiatsu acts on the subtle anatomy of the body described as *qi* in Chinese or *ki* in Japanese. The concept of *qi* might be a bit difficult to grasp at first as it is so little recognized in Western society, but everyone can learn how to perceive *qi* and appreciate its effects. *Qi* is a fundamental idea to Oriental medical thinking and is considered as our "life essence" which maintains and nurtures our physical body

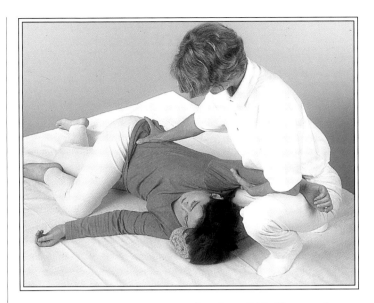

ABOVE: Here the practitioner stretches the gall bladder meridian and opens the rib cage.

and therefore also affects our mind and spirit. *Qi* is everywhere. It moves and changes quickly from moment to moment and can easily be replenished on a day-to-day basis. The human body is a field of continually moving energy, circulating through cells, tissues, muscles and internal organs.

The concept of *qi* was introduced to the West through acupuncture and the Chinese martial art of T'ai Chi Chuan. The Chinese word *qi* translates as "breaths". A Japanese dictionary defines *qi* as mind, spirit, or heart and lists hundreds of expressions which use the word *qi*, most of them ordinary ways of talking about human moods, attitudes, or character. For example, *genki* means "source of *qi*" or health.

It is much easier to demonstrate *qi* than to try to measure or contain it and there are a variety of exercises you can do to get in touch with *qi* and feel its affect on your body. *Qi* is a real force, made up of electric, magnetic, infrasonic and infra-red vibrations, which can be intuitively perceived and mentally directed. Like air that we breathe and depend on for our life and water that we take into our bodies, *qi* is the very source of our vitality. It is the force within us which gives us initiative, which drives and inspires us to move forward in life. When the *qi* leaves us, we die. According to the ancient philosophers, life and death is nothing but an aggravation and dispersal of *qi*:

"*Qi* produces the human body just as water becomes ice. As water freezes into ice, so *qi* coagulates to form the human body. When ice melts, it becomes water. When a person dies, he or she becomes spirit (*shen*) again. It is called spirit, just as melted ice changes its name to water."

WANG CHONG, AD 27–97

THE MERIDIAN LINES

LUNG:
Official in charge of jurisdiction.

The lungs govern *qi* and respiration and in particular are in charge of inhaling air. Intake of fresh *qi* from the environment which is fundamental for building up resistance against external intrusions.

Elimination of gases through the process of exhalation.

Openness and positivity.

LARGE INTESTINE:
Official generating elimination and exchange.

Helps the function of the lungs. Elimination of waste products from food and drink and stagnated *qi*. Transmission.

The ability to let go.

SPLEEN:
Official in charge of storage.

Transformation and nourishment. Spleen corresponds to the function of the pancreas in Western terms and governs general digestion including saliva and gastric bile; secretions from the small intestines; reproductive hormones related to the breasts and ovaries.

Maintains the health of the flesh, the connective soft tissue and the muscle.

Self-image is affected strongly by the spleen function and the desire to help others is apparent. Self-confidence.

STOMACH:
Official in charge of the granary or food store.

The stomach is responsible for receiving and processing ingested food and fluids.

Information for mental and physical nourishment.

Well grounded, centred and reliable.

HEART:
Minister of the monarch and has insight and understanding.

Governs blood and blood vessels.

Houses the mind and our emotions. The heart functions as the mechanism that adapts and integrates external stimuli to the body's internal environment.

Awareness and communication. Joyful.

SMALL INTESTINE:
Official in charge of the treasury who converts food into energy.

The quality of the blood and tissue reflects the condition of the small intestine. Anxiety, emotional excitement or nervous shock can adversely affect the energy of the small intestine.

Emotional stability and calmness.

KIDNEY:
Official who does energetic work.

Provides and stores fundamental *qi* for all other organs and governs birth, growth, reproduction and development.

Nourishes the spine, the bones and the brain.

Vitality, direction and will-power.

BLADDER:
Official in charge of storage of the overflow and fluid secretions.

Purification and regulation.

Gives courage and ability to move forward in life.

HEART GOVERNOR:
Official of joy and pleasure.

Protector of the heart and closely related to emotional responses.

Related to central circulation.

Influences relationships with others.

TRIPLE HEATER:
Official who plans construction.

Transportation of energy, blood and heat to the peripheral parts of the body.

Helpful and emotionally interactive.

LIVER:
Official in charge of planning.

Storage of blood.

Ensures free flow of *qi* throughout the body.

Creative and full of ideas.

GALL BLADDER:
Official with good judgement and decisions.

Stores bile produced by the liver and distributes it to the small intestine.

Practical application of ideas and decision-making.

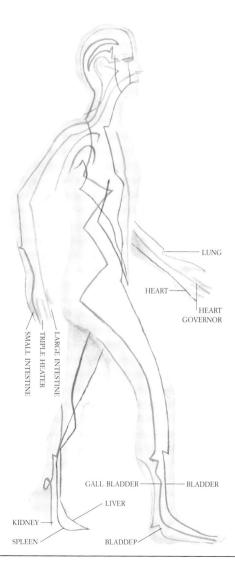

LEFT: Shiatsu works on the body's natural meridians, shown in this diagram. A shiatsu practitioner will work on these lines to promote balance and harmony.

THE MERIDIAN SYSTEM

Each of the twelve organs is linked with a meridian or channel of energy, named according to the internal organ it affects. The meridians connect all the different body parts with each other and like rivers of energy, ensure proper nurturing of *qi* or life force throughout your whole being. When you are healthy, the flow of *qi* proceeds unimpeded, like the water in a free-running river, and energy is well distributed throughout the meridian pathways. When the river, or meridian, is blocked for some reason, the *qi* is prevented from reaching the specific area it is supposed to nurture and cells, tissue or organs will suffer from lack of it.

The area or internal organ/system connected to this meridian will enter a state of "dis-ease", or a condition of stress. In the early stages the symptoms might be minor, perhaps just a nagging pain or discomfort. This is your body telling you that something is wrong.

Any type of "disease" is a sign that the energy within the meridian system is out of balance. When a meridian is blocked, one part of the body is getting too much *qi* and enters a state of excess, while another part is getting too little and becomes deficient in *qi*. This will result in one organ becoming overactive while another organ will become underactive and may be fatigued. If you do not listen to what your body is telling you at this stage, the symptoms might worsen and become more serious – from here degeneration of the system and body begins.

Along the meridians you will find more highly charged energy points, which are called pressure points in English or *tsubo* in Japanese. This is where the *qi* is most easily affected and stimulating different *tsubo* will correct the energy imbalance. By using different shiatsu techniques, such as pressure, stretching, rubbing and corrective exercises, you will be able to release the blockages, "open" the meridian and recharge yourself.

All the meridians either start or end in the hands or the feet and connect internally to the organ whose condition they reflect. Refer to the meridian line illustration for the pathways of the different meridians over the surface of the body and to the table for the functions of the meridians. In Oriental medicine, the organs are thought of in a conceptual sense, with official duties as in a government. When the different "officials" work together and co-operate, there is peace and harmony in the land (body). If there is disagreement or disorganization between the different departments, imbalances start to occur.

A further eight extraordinary meridians known as vessels also carry energy through our bodies. The two most important in their influence as regards shiatsu are the governing vessel and the conception vessel. These vessels are responsible for the control and regulation of the energy circulating throughout the meridian system and any necessary adjustments are made to them when excesses or deficiencies in the energy system occur.

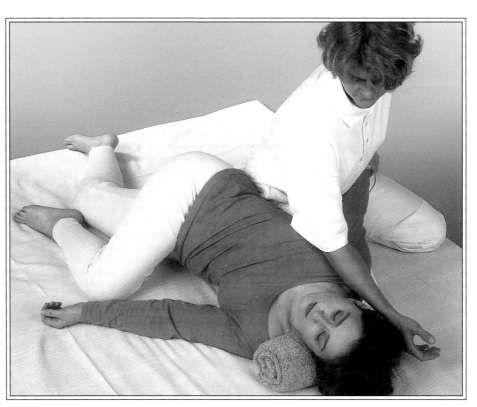

RIGHT: The side position is a classic position used in shiatsu; here the practitioner half kneels beside the patient and opens the chest by gently stretching the lung meridian in the arm.

SHIATSU WITH A PRACTITIONER

A shiatsu session usually lasts for about an hour with the actual treatment taking between 35 and 45 minutes.

In the first session the shiatsu practitioner will ask you many questions about your state of health, your lifestyle, any symptoms, likes and dislikes you may have, to build up your case history. An assessment based on Oriental diagnosis will be compiled. Apart from this oral diagnosis, your practitioner will use visual diagnosis, looking at posture, movement and facial diagnostic areas; and touch diagnosis, feeling the body and the different meridians for areas of excess and deficiency. As touch is the most essential aspect of shiatsu, this diagnosis continues throughout the whole treatment, your practitioner gaining new information about you as the sessions proceed.

You will usually remain clothed during treatment, but your practitioner may need to examine skin surfaces for discolorations and/or swelling at some stage. As the treatment will involve stretches and different movements for you to practise in between sessions, it is advisable to wear loose, comfortable clothing, preferably of cotton. Avoid receiving shiatsu after you have eaten. Digestion will draw energy to the abdomen and disturb your practitioner in reading the energetic movements in your meridian system. There should be as little outside disturbance as possible to maintain the balancing effects of the treatment. It is also suggested therefore that you refrain from consuming any alcohol on the day

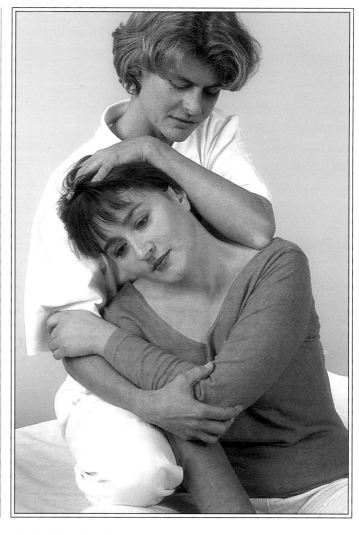

ABOVE: The sitting position is one of the different positions used in a shiatsu treatment. In a supportive way the practitioner is treating the trapezius muscle, affecting the large intestine and gall bladder meridian on top of the shoulder.

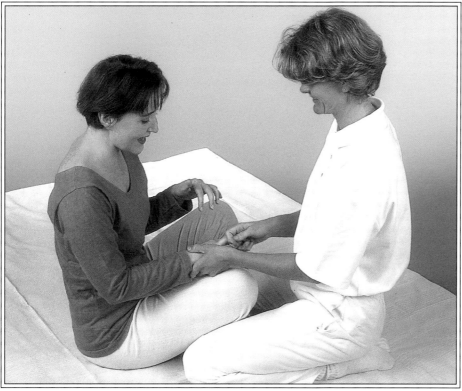

LEFT: All meridians – or energy channels – either start or end in the fingers and toes.

before your treatment as well as the actual day and avoid strenuous exercise following your shiatsu session.

HOW MANY SESSIONS?

A course of treatment usually involves four to eight sessions, preferably on a weekly basis. This depends on the nature of the problem. A long-term imbalance might need more treatments, while a couple of sessions for an acute disturbance might be sufficient. Remember that shiatsu is also a preventive therapy, aiding the maintenance of good health, so you do not need to be unwell to receive treatments. This is why many clients continue their shiatsu sessions, after the initial course of treatments, every month or two for their general health and well-being.

BELOW: Here the practitioner is treating the bladder meridian in the back of the leg, using the knee.

EFFECTS AFTER YOUR SHIATSU TREATMENT

The immediate effect of treatments differs with each individual. Depending on your state of health, your symptoms and how accustomed you are to receiving bodywork, you will have different reactions after your shiatsu treatments. A sense of well-being is common.

Because of the deep relaxation that usually occurs and the stimulus to the major body systems, you may have some healing reactions. Some people feel cold or flu-like symptoms, aches and pains, or headaches after the first treatment. These symptoms will only last for a day or so and usually subside with each subsequent treatment. It is important to remember that any such effects you may experience are positive signs from your body telling you it is making an attempt to correct its own condition in a natural way. These are signs of elimination and the beginning of the healing process.

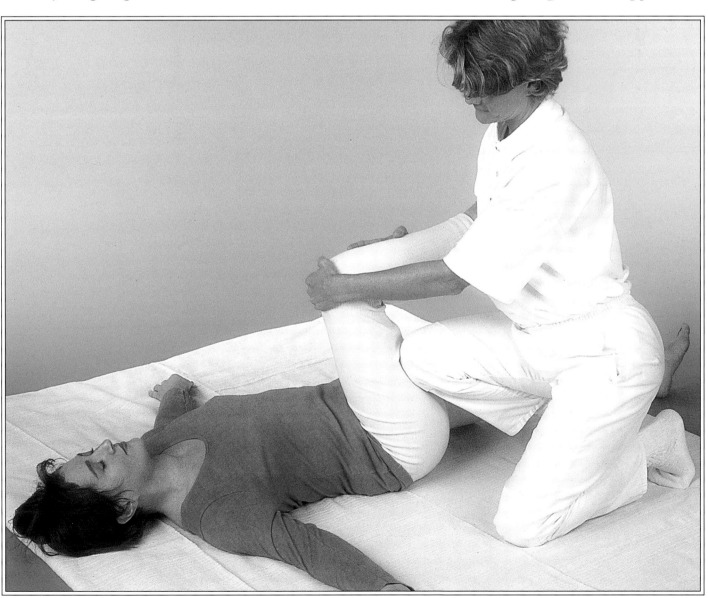

SHIATSU WITH A PARTNER

Here are some simple shiatsu techniques which you can perform on a partner. This is an ideal way to release tension
without putting too much strain on the body. You may feel
sleepy afterwards. Keep your touch gentle.

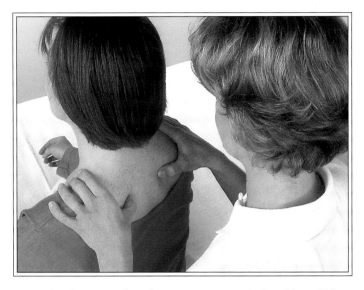

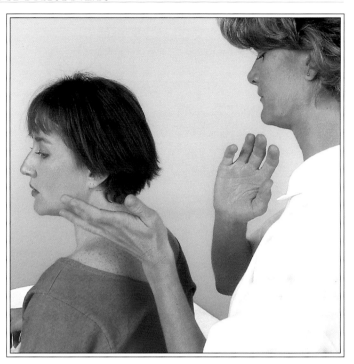

1 Gently place your hands on your partner's shoulders. Take
a moment to tune into her energy. There may be tension in
the area to begin with. Squeeze the trapezius muscle – the
muscles of the shoulder and neck – using your thumbs and
fingers in a rhythmic kneading action.

2 With the little finger side of your hand, gently hack across
the shoulders and neck in a rhythmic motion. Gradually your
partner's muscles will relax and you can increase the intensity
and power of the hacking. Keep checking if this feels
comfortable for your partner.

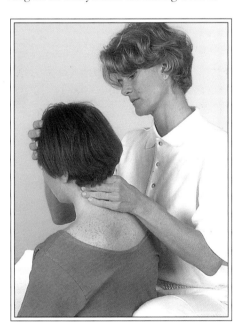

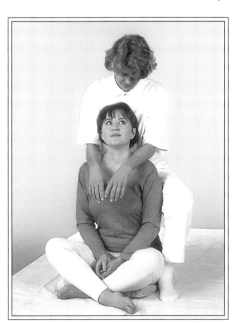

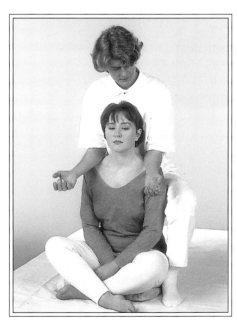

3 Kneel at your partner's side supporting
the back with your leg. Place one hand
on the forehead and encourage the
partner to relax the head into your hand.
With the fingers and thumb of the other
hand, gently squeeze the neck muscles.

4 Kneel behind your partner and place
your forearms on the shoulders with
your palms facing to the floor. Lean into
your forearms using your body to apply
equal gentle pressure on to your
partner's shoulders.

5 Ask your partner to breathe deeply.
On the out breath, roll your arms across
the shoulder, from the neck towards the
shoulder joint, ending up with your
palms facing up. Lift your arms up and
repeat several times.

PRONE POSITION

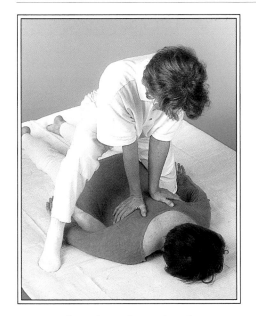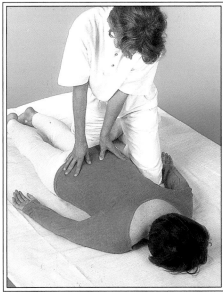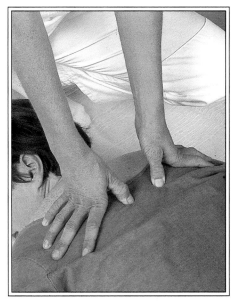

1 Using the palms of your hands, press down gently on your partner's back. Start at the top of the back in between the shoulders and gradually work downwards. Apply the pressure as your partner breathes out. Keep your elbows straight. Repeat three times.

2 Measure two fingers' breadth from the centre of the spine to locate the bladder meridian. Use your thumbs and apply gentle pressure all the way down the back, working gradually from the top to the bottom.

3 For the upper part of the back, kneel or crouch at your partner's head. Using your thumbs, apply pressure to the bladder meridian. Hold this gentle pressure for a few seconds.

COMPLETION

To complete the session, lie your partner down on the back. Rest your hand on the stomach. This is called the Hara in the Orient, and is thought of as the vital centre of ourselves. In this position "tune in" to your partner's breathing. Stay in this position for a few moments until you can sense that your partner is relaxed and peaceful, then slowly move your hand away and gently dissolve the contact.

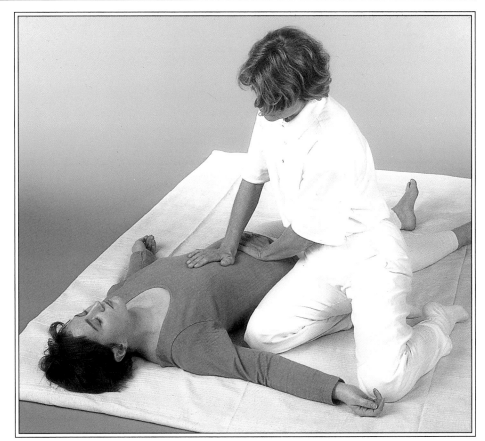

MERIDIAN STIMULATION

The following DoIn (a form of shiatsu) exercises are designed to improve, maintain and develop your general physical, mental and emotional health and well-being.

The exercises can be practised by anyone maintaining a normal daily life, at any time without any special effort. The DoIn exercises will open up the energy channels, release any blockages and facilitate the free flow of *qi* along the meridians, thus improving the circulation of energy throughout the whole body. You will feel invigorated and energized after performing the exercises, and it is recommended that you do them upon rising in the morning, or whenever you are feeling low and generally under par.

Although any part of the series of exercises can be practised independently, it is best to perform the whole sequence at one time to achieve the maximum benefit. Keep a natural posture and breathe normally throughout the exercises and try to maintain an empty mind, clear from any disturbing thoughts and feelings. Keep your focus on the exercise and feel the effect it has on your body. As you become accustomed to the routine, it will be easier to follow and you will find it takes even less time to complete.

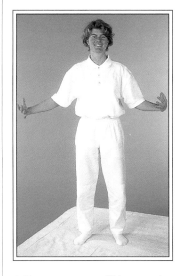

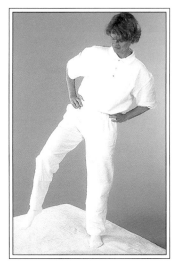

1 Prepare yourself by gently shaking your body. Shake your arms and hands. Lift your shoulders up to your ears as you breathe in; let them relax on exhaling. Repeat a few times.

2 One at a time, gently shake each of your legs and feet. Then sit down in a chair or on a cushion on the floor, keeping your back straight. Keeping an upright posture allows a good energy flow.

HEAD

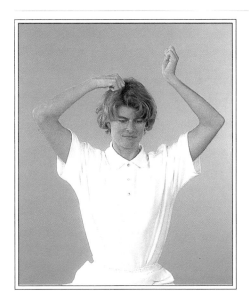

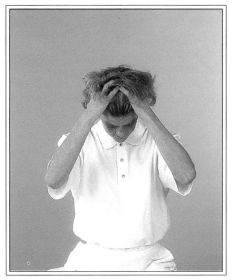

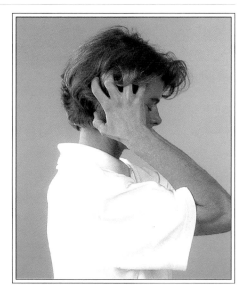

1 Clench both hands loosely and, with your wrists loose, start to tap the top of your head gently. Work your way slowly all around your head, covering the sides, front and back. Adjust the percussion pressure as needed. This exercise will wake up your brain and stimulate blood circulation which will be beneficial for your hair growth and hair quality.

2 Pull your fingers through your hair, gently stimulating the meridians running across the top and side of your head (bladder and gall-bladder).

3 Place your fingers on either side of the mid-line of your skull and apply pressure with your fingertips to the bladder meridian, working from the forehead to the back of your neck. Then move your fingers down to just above the ears and apply pressure. Repeat this sequence three times.

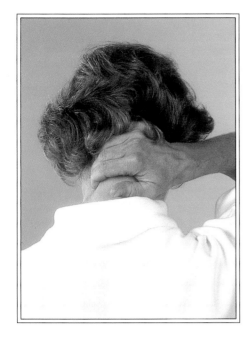

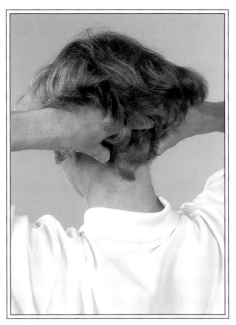

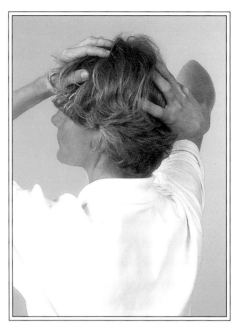

1 Now move your attention to the back of your neck. Bend your head down and using one hand, place your palm across the back of your neck and gently massage it using a squeezing motion.

2 Lift your chin slightly and with your thumbs, press either side of the base of the skull, supporting your head with your fingers. The pressure should be directed up against the skull.

3 Use one thumb to stimulate the skull's mid-base, while the other hand supports your forehead, tipping the head slightly up and back. Vibrate your thumb gently as you apply pressure, then release. Repeat three to five times.

FACE

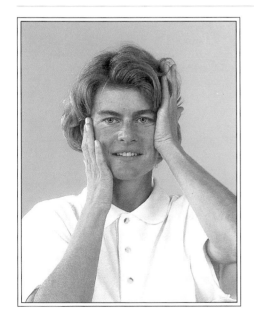

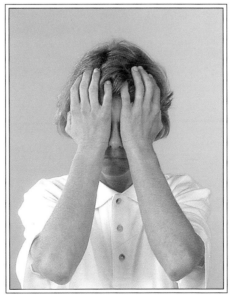

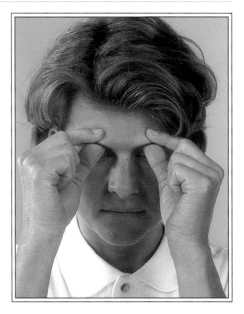

1 Apply both hands to your cheeks and using the palms gently rub your cheeks in an up-and-down motion until the skin becomes warm.

2 Bring your palms to your eyes, covering them and warming the area around the eyes. This stimulates blood circulation in the area and will be beneficial for tired eyes.

3 Using your index finger and thumb, squeeze your eyebrows starting from the centre line and moving laterally, three times.

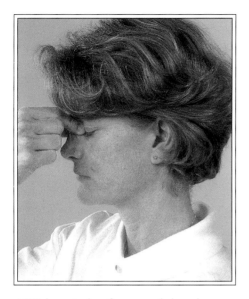

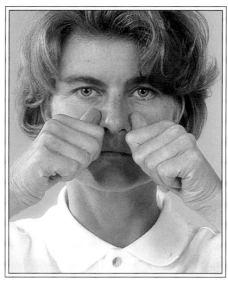

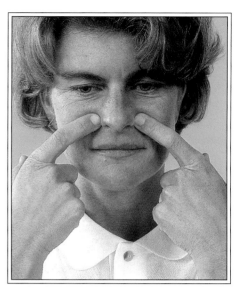

4 With an index finger and thumb, pinch the bridge of the nose and the corners of the eyes. This point is called "eye's clarity". It opens and brightens the eyes and clears vision and will be especially helpful if the eyes are tired.

5 Clench your fingers and apply your thumbs to the sides of your nose. Stroke down the side of your nose quickly at the same time as you breathe in. This will help to clear your sinuses and release any stagnation of mucus.

6 Use your index fingers to stimulate either side of the nose.

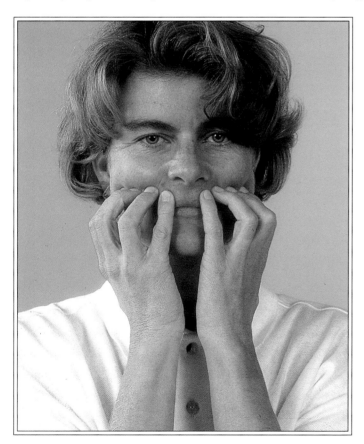

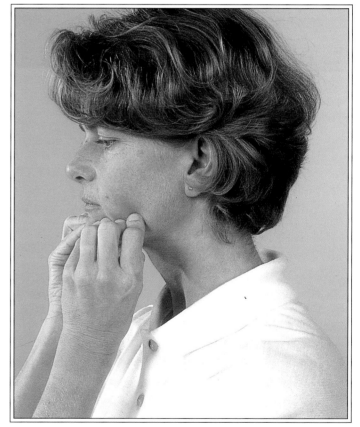

7 Using the four fingers of both hands, apply pressure around the mouth. This area of your face reflects the digestive system and these exercises will activate the production of saliva and strengthen the system.

8 Using your thumbs and index fingers, squeeze your lower jaw. Repeat three to five times. This will stimulate the glands which are directly related to the ears, saliva and lymph so that they function properly.

EARS

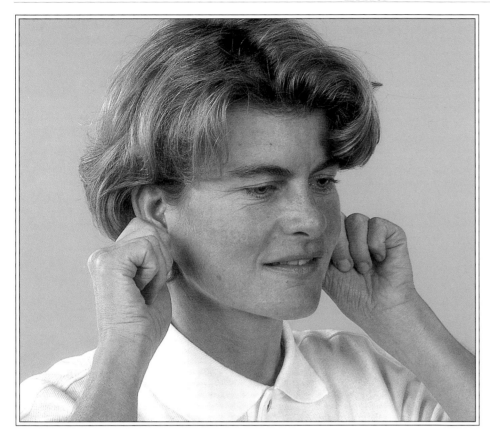

1 Move your hands to your ears and massage them gently, using your index fingers and thumbs. Your ears relate to your kidneys and these exercises will improve mental balance as well as kidney and excretory functions. First rub the peripheral ridge of the ear in order to activate circulation; then rub the middle ridge and finally move to the inner ridges and indentations.

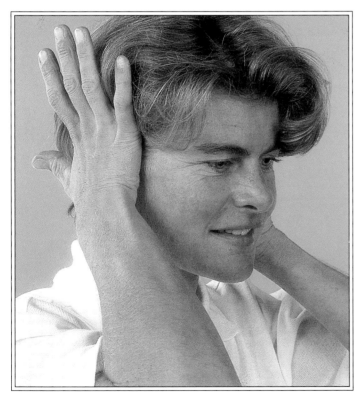

2 Squeeze your ear lobes and then, with the palms of your hands, vigorously rub the whole of both ears, up and down, until they become warm.

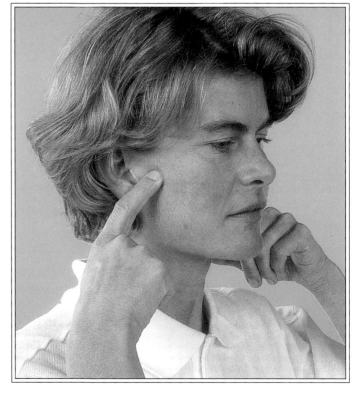

3 If you have a ringing in the ears, apply gentle pressure to the point in front of the middle of the ear.

SHOULDERS AND ARMS

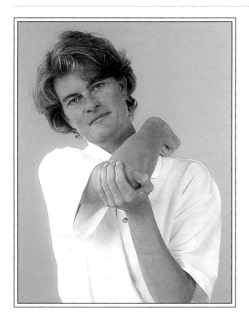

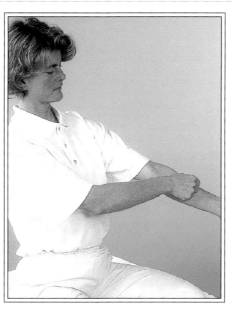

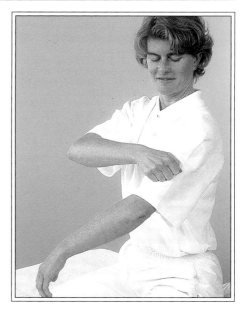

1 Using your left hand to support the right elbow, with a loose fist tap across the top of your left shoulder with your right hand and, as far as you can, reach over your shoulder-blade.

2 Release the elbow, straighten your left arm in front of you, open up your palm and tap down the inside of your arm from the shoulder to the open hand. This will stimulate the energy flow of the lung, heart governor and heart meridians.

3 Turn your arm over and tap up the back of your arm, from the hand back to the shoulder again. This will stimulate the meridians on the back of your arm, namely the large intestine, triple burner and small intestine. Repeat three times.

HANDS

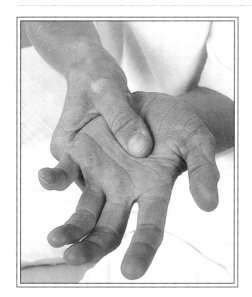

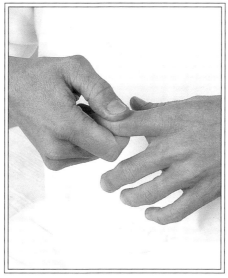

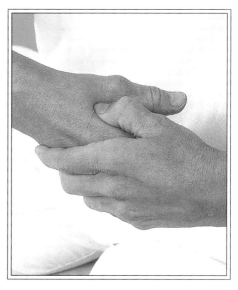

1 Use your right hand to work your left, massaging the centre of your palm gently with your right thumb. The point here is called "palace of anxiety", heart governor 8, and is good for relieving general tension.

2 Rotate and massage the joints of each finger using your right index finger and thumb. This is a great way to release any tension in your hands and helps to prevent arthritis as well as improving flexibility in the joints.

3 Apply pressure in between your thumb and finger. This point will help to relieve headaches, constipation or diarrhoea. It is a point sometimes used to expedite labour; therefore it should not be stimulated during pregnancy.

CHEST AND ABDOMEN

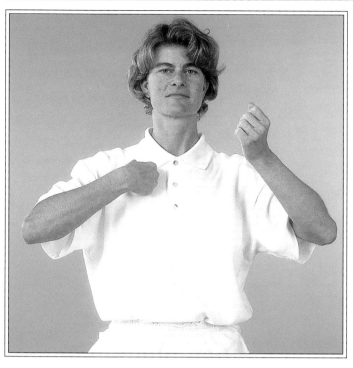

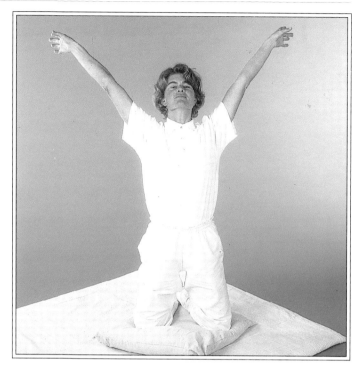

1 Open up your chest by tapping across it with loose fists, above and around your breasts and across the ribs. This will stimulate your lungs and enhance and strengthen your respiratory system.

2 Take a deep breath in as you throw your arms up over your head. Repeat the tapping. This is good for releasing tension in your chest and supporting you in expressing your thoughts and feelings.

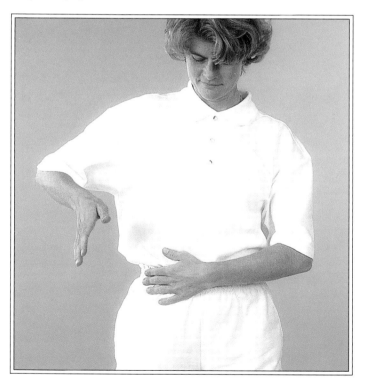

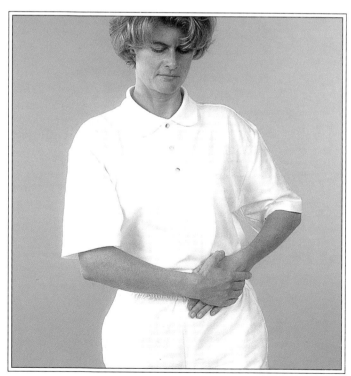

3 Proceed down towards your abdomen and with open hands tap around your abdomen gently in a clockwise direction, going down on the left and up on the right side. This follows the flow of circulation and digestion.

4 Place one hand on top of the other and make the same circular motion around your abdomen for a minute.

BACK

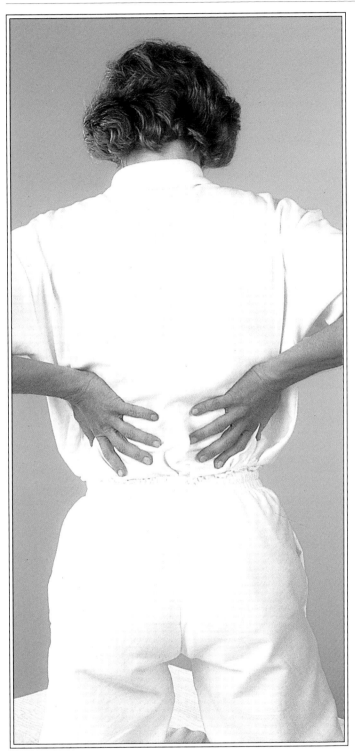

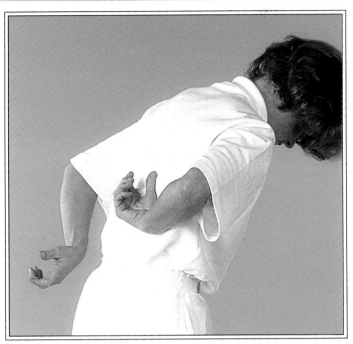

2 Stand up with your feet shoulder-width apart. Bend forward slightly and tap your lower back gently using your loose fists. Reach up as far as possible and move down to the lower part of your spine, your hips and the muscles of your buttocks. Releasing tension in this area will stimulate your digestive and elimination organs.

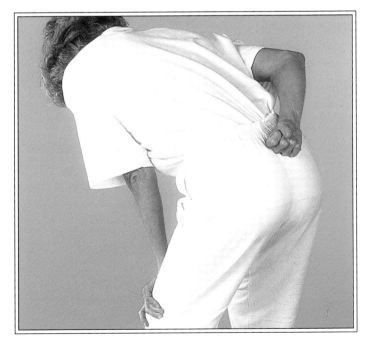

1 Place your hands on your back, just below the rib cage. This is the area of your kidneys. Start to rub the area slowly until you feel some warmth building up under your hands. This stimulates your kidney energy responsible for your vitality and also for warming your body.

3 Using the back of your hand, tap across the sacrum bone at the base of your spine. This activates your nervous system and sends energy vibrations up the spine to your brain. Tapping the coccyx also decongests the sinuses, so breathe deeply through the nose when practising this exercise.

LEGS AND FEET

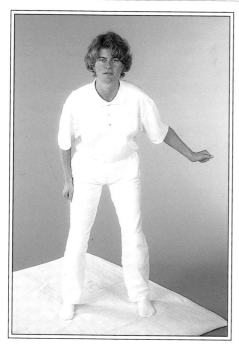

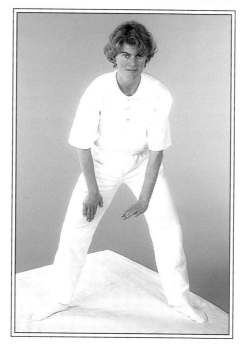

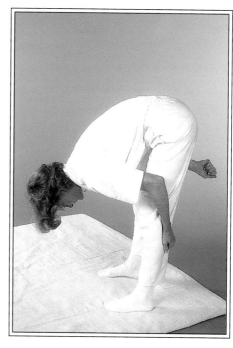

1 Stand with your feet wider apart. Keeping your knees slightly bent, start tapping with your fists down the outside of your legs from the hips to your ankles. This is where your gall-bladder meridian is located.

2 Now tap up the inside of your legs from the ankle to the groin area, stimulating your liver and spleen meridians. Use the palms of your hand rather than a fist if you prefer.

3 Then tap down the back of your legs following the flow of energy in your bladder meridian, from your buttocks to your heels. Come up the inside of your legs again.

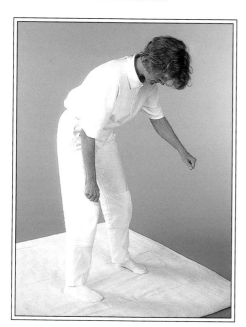

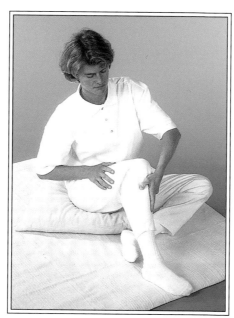

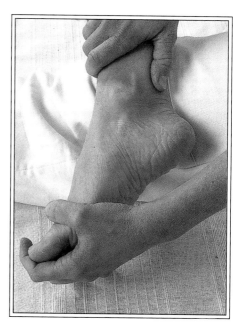

4 Tap down the front of your legs, slightly outside the big quadriceps muscle. Tap all the way down to the front of your ankles and then come up the inside of your legs. Repeat this whole sequence three times.

5 Along the stomach meridian there is a good point for general well-being, on the outside of your leg, below your knee. Apply gentle pressure for a few seconds.

6 Remain seated on the floor, hold your foot and make a circular movement at the ankle to free up joint mobility.

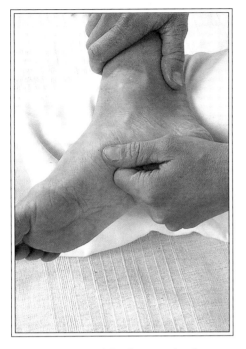

7 Tap the sole of the foot, with a loose fist, then massage the whole foot with both hands.

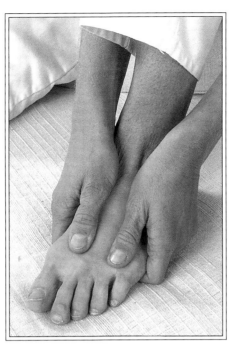

8 Hold your hands under the bottom of your foot and use your thumbs to rub downward along the top of your foot, in between each metatarsal bone to your toes.

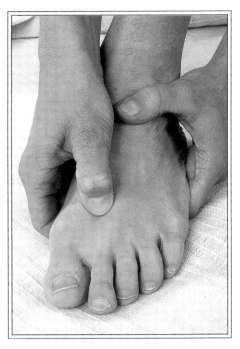

9 Massage the web between each toe and then massage the toe joints gently. The point between the big toe and the second toe is good for abdominal cramps: do not use during pregnancy.

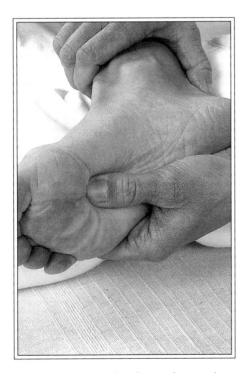

10 Come to the sole of your foot and apply pressure to this point with your thumb. This will have a revitalizing effect upon your body and stimulate energy flow.

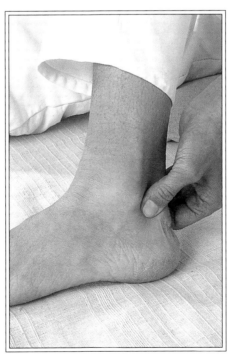

11 Use your thumbs to massage the area under the ankle bone. This area, spleen 6, located four fingers' width up from the inside ankle bone, is a great point to use for any menstrual disorders.

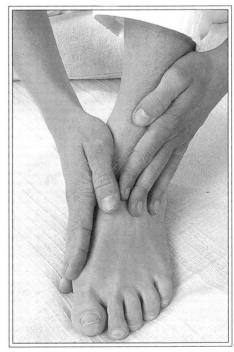

12 Give the whole foot a good rub. Then grab hold of your ankle with both hands and shake out your foot. Now repeat this whole sequence with your other foot.

COMPLETION

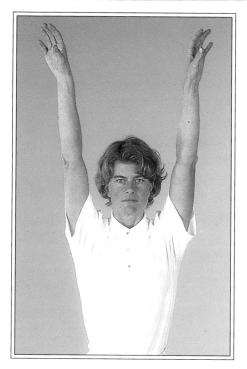

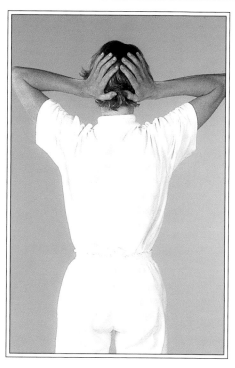

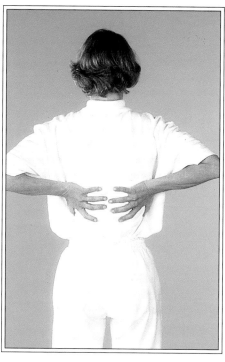

1 After having worked your body, stroke your meridians gently. First stand up with your feet apart. Take a deep breath in and lift your arms up.

2 As you breathe out, bend your arms and place your hands on your head. Stroke down the back of your head to your neck.

3 Bring your hands as high up as possible underneath the shoulder-blades and stroke down the whole of your back, buttocks and legs.

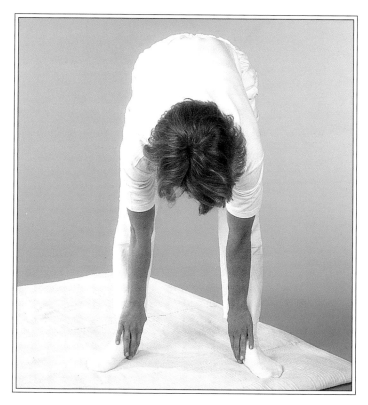

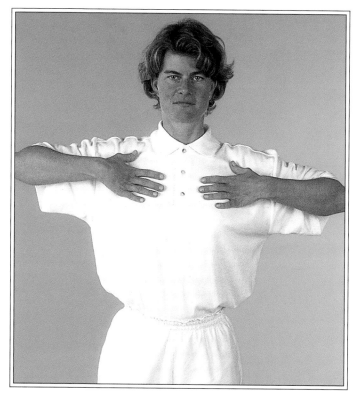

4 Open your legs and come up the inside of your legs to the groin area. Proceed up the front over your abdomen and up to your chest.

5 Stroke out to the sides and open up your chest. Open your arms to the sides and then repeat the whole completion sequence again, three to five times.

MAKKO HO

The makko ho exercises originated in Japan and were developed to improve the flow of energy or *qi* in our bodies. They are widely used in the shiatsu world as a self-healing technique for practitioners and clients alike. Each exercise works on a specific pair of meridians, enhancing their function, and the full sequence of six exercises covers the whole body and its organs.

In makko ho you will find references in the text to the five Chinese elements of earth, fire, water, wood and metal. These elements are used in Oriental medicine for diagnosis, and even in the West we use expressions such as "he's all fired-up", or "she's very wooden" (meaning very stiff).

Where you find an element mentioned, try to think of its quality – the warmth and vitality of fire, the clear purifying aspect of free-flowing water, the strength and flexibility of wood, the firmness of the earth, the fine quality of air at the top of a mountain. The qualities of air are included in the metal element. Use your imagination and you will discover the elemental qualities in yourself.

When carried out regularly and with correct attention, the exercises serve as an excellent self-diagnostic tool and also enable people to improve not only the function of their organs but also their emotional and psychological states, which relate to and are governed by their meridians.

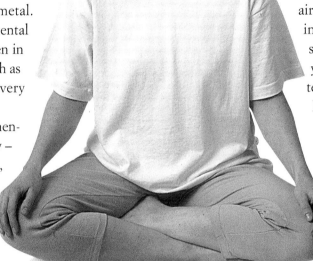

ABOVE: When practising makko ho exercises, focus your attention on your breathing and on the way it changes.

ATTITUDE AND BREATHING

While carrying out the makko ho exercises it is important to note that they will be less effective if their form is merely copied – even though the body will be well stretched. The true benefits of these exercises will be properly discovered by exploring them with the right level of attention.

The whole point of the makko ho exercises is to really feel into them and to use your breath to bring an awareness to the changing sensations in your body as you move through them.

Breathing is the vital focus which enables you to work with your body's limitations and to encourage change in its habitual functioning. Throughout the exercises be aware of the qualities of each breath that you take.

As you breathe in, the body fills up with air and expands and there is a natural increased tension as everything stretches. You can then observe how your body responds to this increased tension. Do you feel that there is any kind of irritation or resistance in your body tissues, or do you feel that they are enjoying the extra stretch – delighting in it, feeling alive and vibrant?

Observe how your mind or emotions respond to the tension. Are you happy and feeling good, or are you feeling angry or sorry for yourself? Note these and any other responses but try not to get trapped in them. Remember to be aware that the exercises and the breathing are enabling you to become more deeply in touch with yourself.

As you breathe out, the body is letting go of air and some waste products, with a physical relaxation in the body tissues. Observe how this affects you. Is there a feeling of relief in your body? How do you feel? Do you feel calmer and more at peace, or sad and experiencing some difficulty in surrendering to the exhaled breath?

At first, when you do the exercises you may find it difficult to think this way, but when you focus your attention on your breathing, you can really begin to discover something about yourself, your body and your reactions to the ever-changing qualities of the inhaled and exhaled breath.

THE PRACTICE OF MAKKO HO EXERCISES

Ideally the makko ho exercises should be practised at least once every day. It is beneficial to practise them on waking in the morning, to ease out the stiffness of sleep gently and to prepare for the day. They may also be done in the evening to refresh oneself after work, or before going to bed to enhance sleep.

It is important to carry out the exercises in the order they are given because this follows the natural flow of energy through the body and its organs. When the *qi,* or life force, is not flowing properly through the body, it becomes stuck or stagnant somewhere and this might lead to disease and illness in time. These exercises will act on the body to disperse the blockages and help the energy to flow unimpeded where it needs to go – nurturing the areas that are depleted

BELOW: It is important in makko ho to ease to your own personal limit gently, without forcing anything. Be kind to yourself.

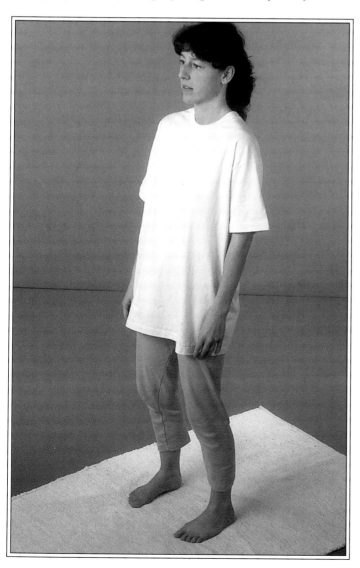

and undernourished and rebalancing your body as a whole.

In order to enhance your body's healing potential through the makko ho exercises and to deepen your understanding of yourself, you should carry out the whole sequence of exercises three times, together with a specific, self-healing phase where you work on two exercises of your own choice.

The optimum practice of the makko ho exercises used here is as follows:

1 Follow the exact sequence of the six exercises as described in detail below. Take your time using your breath and focused attention and do each exercise three times before moving on to the next one. This first series helps to stretch the physical body and disperse tension.

2 Repeat the whole sequence and this time bring more awareness to how you feel in your mind and body as you breathe through the exercises. Note which exercise you feel really comfortable with and would like to stay in for a long time; and which you strongly dislike or have most resistance to.

3 Self-healing phase:

(i) Choose the exercise that you liked best and do it once slowly and stay in the position, breathing and relaxing into it and feeling nurtured by it. By focusing in this way you help to draw energy gently to where it is needed and this will affect your mind and emotions as well as your body. When you feel ready, come slowly out of the position and pause.

(ii) The second choice you now make helps to balance your overall energy pattern. Choose the exercise you least liked, the one in which you felt very tense or irritable. Work more quickly with this one, without straining, and repeat it again and again using the exhaled breath to help you release tension, until you begin to feel tired or easier with the exercise. This method will help to disperse excess energy where it was blocked or sticking, thus allowing a freer flow again.

4 Repeat the whole sequence of exercises once more and note any changes in yourself, in your sensations or attitude as you move through them.

5 Rest on the floor for a few minutes to allow your body to assimilate and settle after the exercises. Breathe gently and deeply without straining and relax.

LUNGS AND LARGE INTESTINE

The lung and large intestine meridians are concerned with exchange of air and elimination of waste products. They represent the metal element which is connected with the air, breathing, boundaries and the emotion of grief. Be especially aware of the breath and the qualities of taking in and letting go in this exercise. Remember to keep observing your sensations and feelings. This exercise will help with breathing problems and regulate elimination.

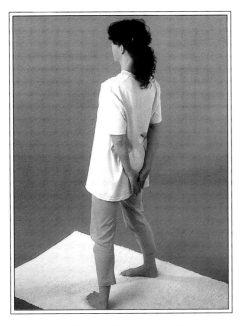

1 Stand with feet shoulder-width apart, toes turned slightly inwards, and feel your connection to the earth. Link your thumbs behind your back and check that your jaw is relaxed.

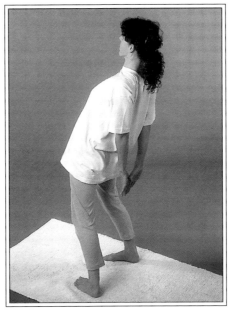

2 Breathe in, feeling the breath fill your body and lungs. Breathe out, straightening your arms, open the chest and lean slightly backwards.

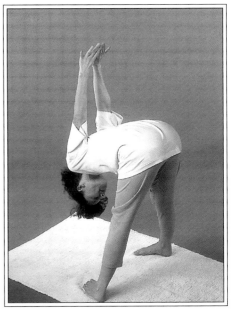

3 Breathe out, bending forward with your back, arms and legs straight. Keep this position for three breaths. On the third exhaled breath, return to your original position. Repeat twice more.

HEART AND SMALL INTESTINE

The heart and small intestine meridians represent the qualities of assimilation of food and integration of external stimuli and emotions in the body. Representing the fire element, they promote warm-heartedness and joy in our lives. Be aware of an alive warmth and increased circulation in this exercise.

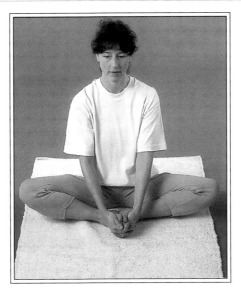

1 Sit on the floor, place the soles of your feet together, hold them and draw them close to your body. Breathe in, feeling a warm expansion in your body.

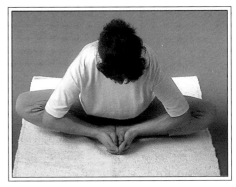

2 On the exhaled breath, draw your body down, bending your elbows and easing your knees towards the floor. Do not strain your hips. Keep your back straight. Breathe fully three times in position, feeling expansion in your back and observe how you feel. On the third exhaled breath, return to the original position. Repeat twice more.

BLADDER AND KIDNEYS

The bladder and kidney meridians relate the water element and qualities of fluidity and easy flow in our lives. Connected to the nervous system, they may become stressed, leading to a fearful state of mind and rigidity in the body. During this exercise concentrate on welcoming the qualities of easy-flowing, purifying water. Imagine it is gently washing over you like a wave, cleansing you and easing away any fears, tension and distress.

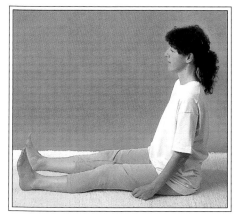

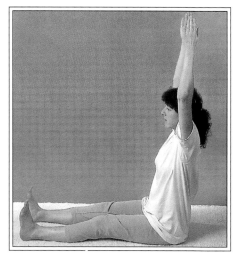

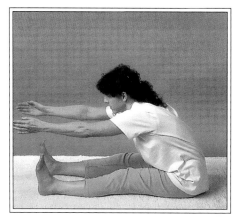

1 Sit upright with your feet parallel, hip-width apart, pointing upwards at a 90° angle to the floor, or towards your head. This will keep your knees straight.

2 On the inhaled breath, draw your arms up above your head, palms facing each other. Keep your back straight.

3 Breathe out and ease forward, bending from the hips, arms forward, parallel to the legs. Look ahead. Ease farther forward on another breath. On the third breath, release the position.

TRIPLE HEATER AND HEART PROTECTOR

The triple heater and heart protector meridians relate to the fire element in its quieter aspect, like a gentle candle flame. They have a protective function in the body on the physical level of immunity and temperature control, and also emotionally – helping us to cope with the knocks and crises in life, especially with regard to relationships.

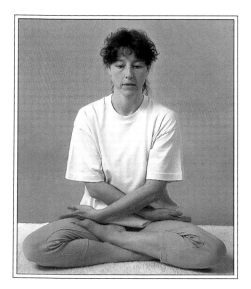

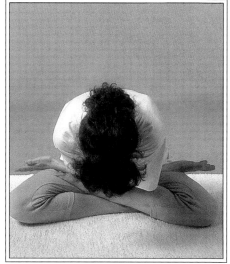

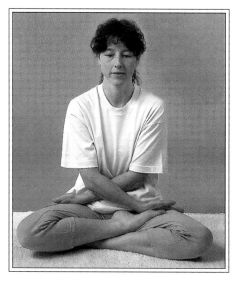

1 Sit, cross-legged, with one or both feet on your thighs. Cross your arms and rest your hands on your thighs, palms facing upwards, fingers together. Do not strain your knees, if you are not comfortable simply cross your legs.

2 Breathe in feeling a warm expansion. On the exhaled breath slide your hands out sideways from the body, keeping your palms flat and horizontal. Bring your body forward, without collapsing.

3 As you breathe three times, feel a warm protection within you. On the third exhaled breath return to the original position. Repeat twice, then cross your legs and arms over the other way and continue three more times.

LIVER AND GALL-BLADDER

The liver and gall-bladder meridians relate to the wood element and the tree's qualities of strength and flexibility when it is healthy. Try to feel these qualities in yourself as you explore this exercise and be aware that when your body feels stiff, you may feel frustrated and angry.

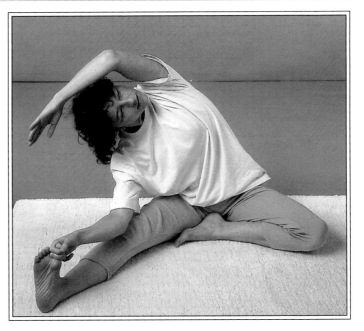

2 On the exhaled breath lean sideways over your right leg grasping your big toe if possible, keeping your leg straight, and easing your body downwards. Do not strain. Keep your chest open and your left arm close to your ear. Feel a strong stretch to the side of your body. Look upwards. Do not collapse your chest or bring your raised arm in front of your face. Breathe three times, inviting the qualities of flexibility into your body and observe how you feel. Release on the third exhaled breath. Repeat three times.

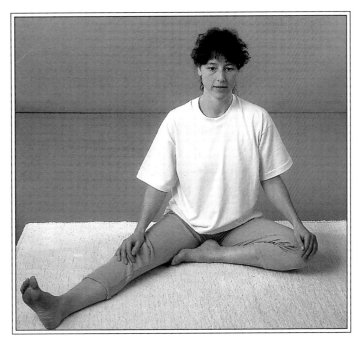

1 Sit upright with your right leg outstretched and flat on the floor; the foot is vertical to keep the knee straight. Tuck your left foot into the body. Breathe in, feeling an alive quality.

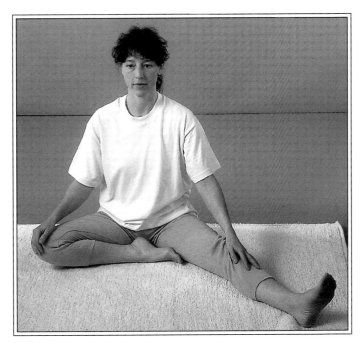

3 Return to the upright position and then change sides with your left leg stretched out and your right foot in. Breathe in.

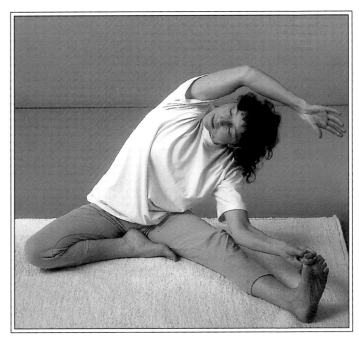

4 On the exhaled breath lean sideways as before, this time to the left. Breathe three times. Repeat three times.

FINISHING EXERCISE

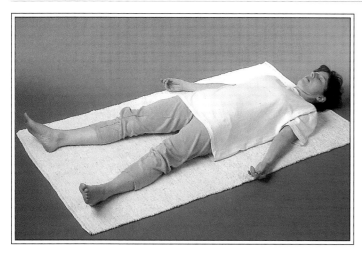

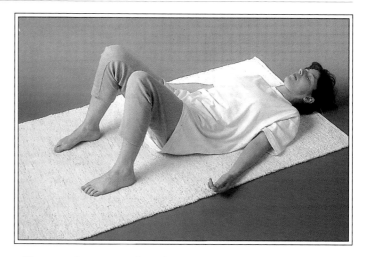

1 After you have completed the whole sequence (ideally three times plus the specific self-healing phase), lie flat on the floor with your eyes closed and just breathe gently for a few minutes, allowing everything to settle in your body.

2 You may be aware of tingling sensations as your inner energy responds to your makko ho exercise session. Another finishing position is lying flat on the floor with your knees up. Breathe into your stomach and relax.

FURTHER PRACTICE
Human nature being what it is, it is inevitable that resistances to doing these exercises will occur at some stage. You are encouraged to note your resistances and continue the exercises anyway and not to give up in the first week, before you really begin to feel the benefits of the makko ho exercises. While acknowledging the hectic pace of our lives, it can always be possible to carry out at least one sequence of exercises per day. Obviously the more time and energy you give to yourself, the greater the benefits will be. May you enjoy your exploration and be well and happy.

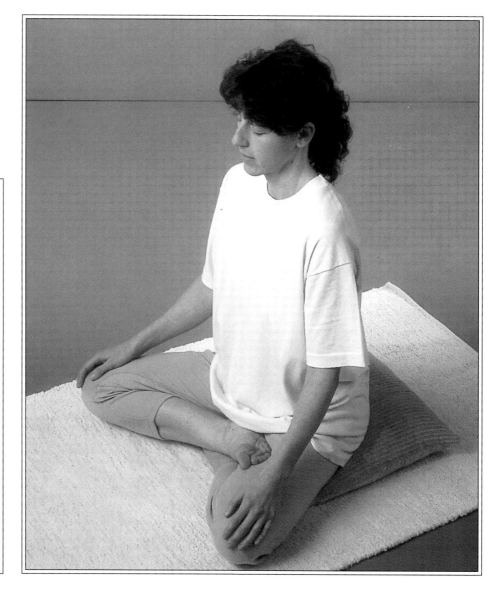

YOGA

The word yoga is by now well known outside India. In fact, over the last four decades it has quietly and steadily taken root in Western culture and language. Yet if you ask a number of people what yoga is, you are likely to get many different responses. These responses are sometimes contradictory. However, yoga can be summarized into the following three possibilities or approaches.

1 YOGA AS POWER

First, yoga can be explained as a means to attain a degree of power or control over the body and mind. Yoga links the body and the mind through intense physical and mental effort. For instance, through rigorous physical practices a state of concentration is developed and maintained which is used to hold power over the body and the breath. Within this approach, such control is often seen as a prerequisite to the body and mind becoming free of disturbances and distractions. This power arises out of three areas of personal development:

> i) Mastery of the body through physical postures;
> ii) Control of the breath through breathing techniques;
> iii) The ability to concentrate through mental techniques.

This intense effort produces energy and control that is available for whatever purpose suits one's direction in life. Many people could usefully enjoy more power over certain areas of their lives. The question is whether they are prepared to put in some effort to reach this point.

In the words of a yoga teacher from long ago: "Yoga is the means by which that which was not attained

RIGHT: Yoga is a process by which you grow in self-understanding.

earlier is now attained." This approach is known as the yoga of energy and will. As such, this aspect of yoga is an art and offers a fascinating field to explore. It appeals to many people searching for power in and over their lives. However, this approach is only a means towards a more important goal.

2 YOGA AS MEDITATION

Here the concern is more with the mystery of life rather than the mastery of life and yoga is a means for meditation with self-inquiry as the primary focus. "Who am I?" is the question that acts as a map for an inner journey into your mind. It is a quest to touch and be touched by the "soulful" quality of being that resides within a person. In this approach, yoga is a tool for a movement towards a deeper relationship with your sense of soul, by searching both into and beyond what you experience as the everyday self. It is a journey of discovery, exploring and ultimately going beyond attitudes that, for better or for worse, have shaped your life, work and relationships.

Yoga is a skill by which you seek to sustain awareness and clarity in spite of the vagaries of everyday life. The quality of this awareness engenders a freshness within which actions are less affected by the usual attitudes and habits. In other words, there is more choice over how you respond or react. In those situations where your reaction would have been automatic, there are now different possibilities.

Yoga is a process by which you grow in your understanding of yourself. From this you come to realize that you can change those aspects of yourself that are unhelpful on your journey through life. This means first recognizing the qualities that hinder your personal growth – an important, if not always comfortable, stage in the journey. Second, having reflected on how you are rather than who you are, you go on to discover that there exists within you a resource with the potential to transform these undesirable aspects. From this you can take steps towards living more creatively. Here again a teacher is important as a guide for advice and suggestions on practices to support the process of growth into an understanding of how you are and ultimately who you are. To quote another saying from the teachings on meditation: "Before I can be nobody, I must first be somebody." This approach is known as the yoga of reflection and discovery.

3 YOGA AS THERAPY

Here, yoga, as both a restorative and preventive, is applied as a therapy to help people with emotional problems or poor health. Here the approach needs to be very different for each person. One person's potential to change his or her situation will be affected by his or her problem, while another person's problem will be affected by his or her potential to change his or her situation.

According to traditional Indian medicine, becoming known in the West as Ayurveda, those diseases that are chronic and cannot be resolved by medicine alone can be helped by using yoga practices. Old yoga texts also talk about the benefits of certain postures and breathing techniques in the treatment of disease.

Using these ideas, it is possible, primarily within a one-to-one relationship, to introduce personalized yoga practices. These practices can both respect the problems or disease in the individual and support his or her intention to influence the way he or she is affected in similar situations in the future.

However, most people experience the dominance of their old ways when confronted with familiar situations. They would like to change but the old patterns are powerful and resist alternatives. It even seems that sometimes what they would really like to do is to carry on exactly as before but without the troublesome symptoms which accompany their lifestyle. To ignore or block these symptoms through

continual suppression will ultimately prove a futile path.

The process of one's inner intelligence is such that it will let one know what needs looking at with increasingly strident messages. This means that the steps to ignore these messages must also intensify. Better to co-operate with yourself before you are forced to by a more serious consequence.

In this respect, yoga as a therapy also presumes that you are willing to accept some responsibility within your situation. Here, with the support of a teacher, you can introduce and work towards sustaining creative changes in your lifestyle. This may also include, as well as specific practices, a review of those relationships which exacerbate your problems. This approach is known as the yoga of rejuvenation and prevention.

YOGA PRACTICES IN THERAPY

The above three aspects of yoga – therapy, power and meditation – are mutually supportive in helping to maintain physical health, psychological vitality and spiritual purpose within the commitments of daily life, work and relationships. The guiding principle is to see the person rather than the problem or disease and to accept that more than a preordained technique is involved. Because of his or her lifestyle, a person may be experiencing certain problems or illnesses. It is also presumed that the situation has become such that the person is willing to explore alternatives to develop a more harmonious relationship between his or her inner nature and outer lifestyle.

ABOVE: At the end of a yoga session you will feel warm, relaxed and alert. Take time to feel these benefits, and to collect your thoughts before you get up.

CHOOSING APPROPRIATE ASANA OR POSTURES

A good starting-point from which to explore yoga is the physical body and the practice of postures which will generate an improvement in the overall function of the system rather than just the form of the body. In yoga these body postures are called "asana" and although many different positions are possible, only a few are required in the area of therapy. Here are six different positions which are not too far from those used in everyday life.

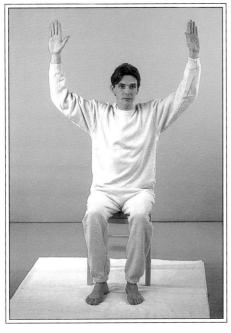

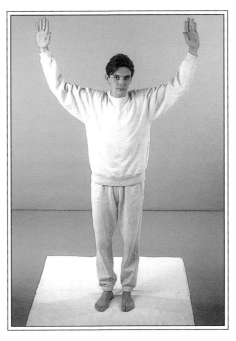

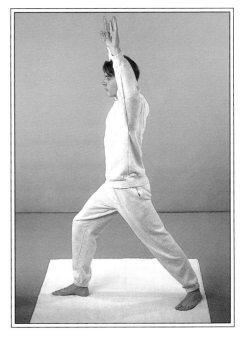

1 A simple starting posture, especially useful if tired. On an inhale, raise your arms, keeping your shoulders relaxed. On the exhale, lower the hands on to the thighs.

2 A similar movement but taken from a standing position. Keep your elbows relaxed, concentrate on allowing the neck to stay tension-free.

3 Another standing posture, this time a more challenging position to stimulate and invigorate. The posture's focus is in the chest and upper back.

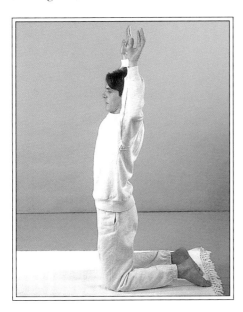

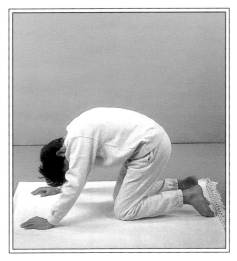

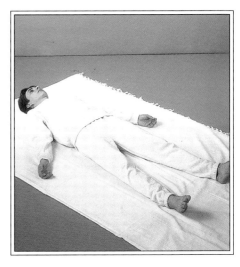

4 A typical kneeling posture, adaptable as either a preparatory movement for other more demanding postures, or a posture for beginners.

5 A kneeling-forward bend is valuable where the back and legs are stiff and as a counterposture to more demanding postures. A good pose for beginners.

6 A lying posture is helpful for rest and relaxation as well as recovery between more demanding postures. A useful pose for all situations and all levels of experience.

MOVEMENT IN ASANA PRECEDES STAYING

The first requirement when using yoga to work with the body within a therapeutic situation is to encourage a creative flow of energy throughout the system. For this, the notion of repeatedly moving into and out of a posture is emphasized rather than holding a posture for a certain amount of time. Here are two sets of repeated movements to try out. When you have developed an ease of practice, the concept of staying and focusing on a particular area can then be considered.

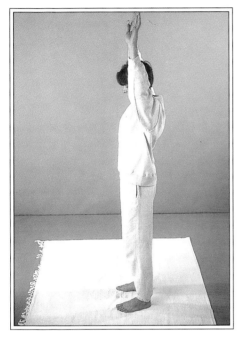

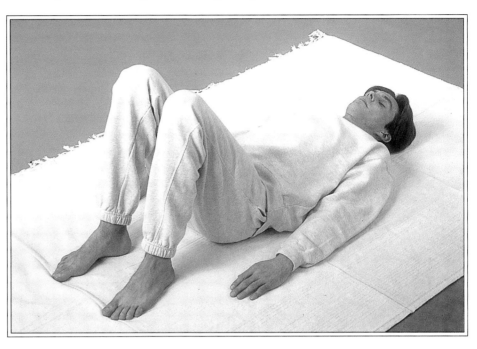

1 Stand with your feet slightly apart and your arms above your head.

1 Lie on your back with your knees bent and your feet flat on the floor. Keep your arms by your sides with the palms facing to the floor. Keep your breathing steady.

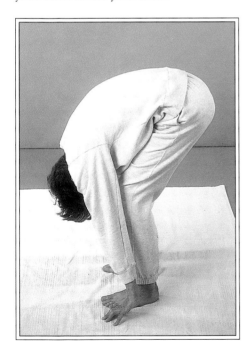

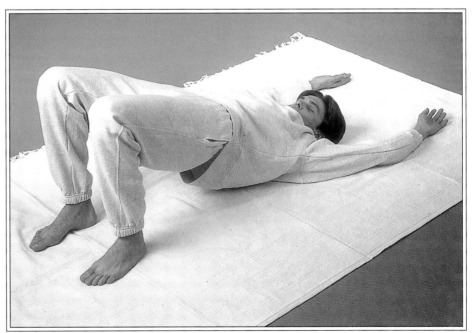

2 Using a slow, unhurried movement, bend at the waist and touch the floor either side of your feet. Bend your legs if you need to. Return to the standing position and repeat.

2 Move your arms so that they are above your head but still resting on the ground, palms facing upwards. Slowly lift your body, with the weight on your feet and shoulders, so that your pelvis is off the ground. Hold for a few seconds, then slowly return to the first position. Repeat.

BREATHING AS AN INTEGRAL PART OF MOVEMENT

To assist in creating a smooth, flowing movement, conscious breathing is added to the movement. This assists a sense of involvement, acts as a measure for anticipating stress and offers a sense of harmony in linking breath, body and mind. Within postures, except when resting, always breathe through the nostrils rather than the mouth. Beginners may find it takes practice to develop correct breathing. Co-ordinate the speed of the movement with the length of your breath. Forward bending or closing movements are generally done with an exhalation, backward bending or opening movements generally with an inhalation.

A ROLE FOR THE MIND IN PRACTICE

These yoga practices need a certain quality of mental concentration, to help steady the body and focus the mind. To help in linking your faculties, you have the rhythm of the movement plus the harmony of the breath to engage your mind. There are also other techniques, such as working with the eyes closed, or counting the length of the breath. As you become more proficient, try these techniques to increase the benefit of the exercises.

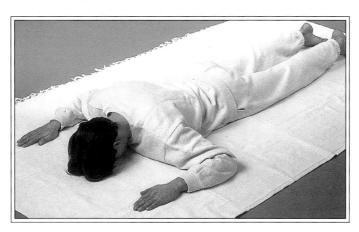

1 Lie on your stomach, face down, with your legs relaxed and slightly apart. Breathe in and allow your chest to lift, keeping your shoulders relaxed.

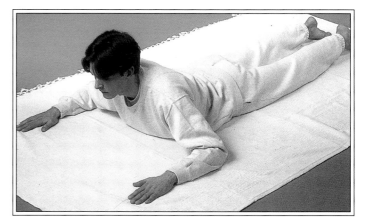

2 Come up as far as you can without straining. Breathe in, wait for a second, and then allow the exhale to bring you slowly back to the starting position. Repeat four to six times.

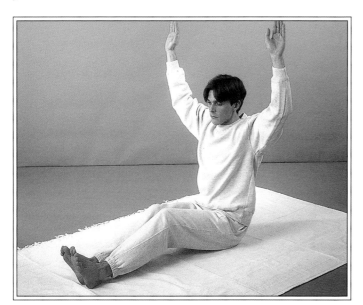

1 Now change your position and sit with your legs extended out in front of you and your knees slightly bent. Breathe in as you lift your arms above your head, keeping the shoulders relaxed. As you breathe out, bend forwards over your knees.

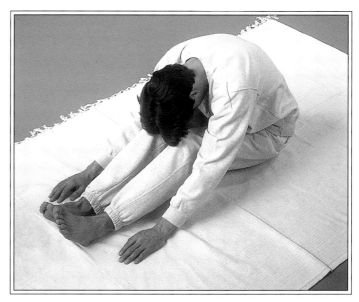

2 As you reach the limit of the exhale, allow your head and shoulders to relax with your hands resting on the ground. Begin to breathe in again, lifting the arms off the ground and sitting up until you have reached the starting position. Start the next exhale and repeat the movement.

ADAPTING THE POSTURE TO THE PERSON

It is also important that the posture is adapted to the person and not the person to the posture. If necessary, the basic posture should be modified to allow access to the form. The bodies of many students, especially in a therapy situation, are limited by age, weight or stiffness.

In yoga terms, the spine is the mainstay of your being at many levels. Therefore anything you do with posture needs to influence your spine, and any adaptations of the postures need to be applied with this in mind. Here are two more postures with alternative adaptations.

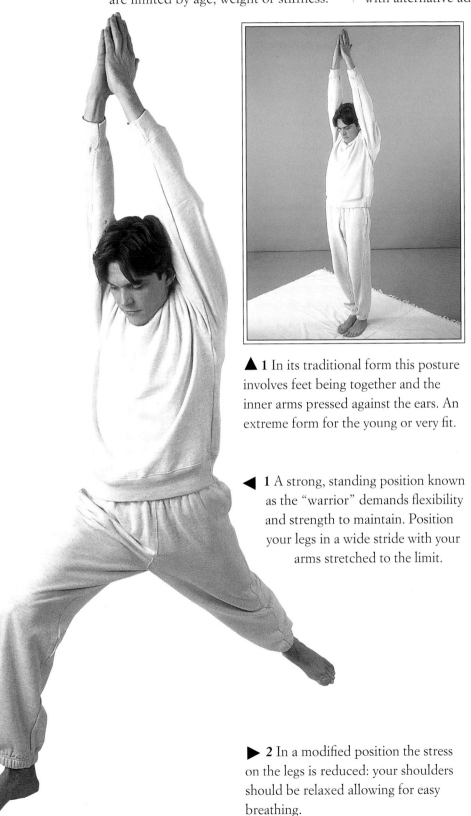

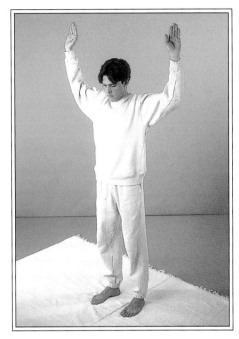

▲ **1** In its traditional form this posture involves feet being together and the inner arms pressed against the ears. An extreme form for the young or very fit.

2 An adaptation offering a more appropriate form for beginners: keep your shoulders relaxed and your chest open to allow free breathing.

◀ **1** A strong, standing position known as the "warrior" demands flexibility and strength to maintain. Position your legs in a wide stride with your arms stretched to the limit.

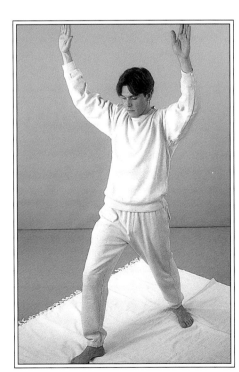

▶ **2** In a modified position the stress on the legs is reduced: your shoulders should be relaxed allowing for easy breathing.

PUTTING THESE PRINCIPLES TOGETHER

These principles introduce the basic guidelines that accompany your first steps into practice. Perhaps it would be helpful at this point to try an experiment aimed at pulling together these different ideas into a personal experience.

Sit comfortably on a chair with your spine erect and unsupported and your hands resting palms down on your thighs. Now go through the following exercises, repeating each set four times only. The actual exercises simply involve raising and lowering the arms. Each set of movements will, however, add a further level of engagement with the intention of deepening your involvement. Here you are inviting an experience of the way that you need to work if yoga is to be effective as a therapy. Focus on the smoothness and length of the breath and the flow of the movements.

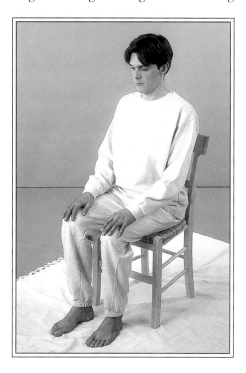

1 Sit on a chair with your spine erect and unsupported and your feet flat on the floor in line with your knees and slightly apart. Rest your hands on your knees with your palms facing downwards.

2 Raise and lower your arms in a forward direction. Repeat this movement four times. Then rest in the first position. Repeat the exercise but this time lower your arms as you breathe out through the nostrils, raising your arms to any breathing pattern you wish. Do this four times.

3 Repeat the exercise. This time raise your arms on the inhalation and lower your arms on the exhalation. Again, breathe through the nostrils rather than the mouth. Now raise and lower your arms as before but consciously lengthen the exhalation while keeping it smooth as you lower your arms.

4 Repeat the process but this time work with your eyes closed. Remember to keep your attention focused on the smoothness and length of the breath as well as the flow of the movements.

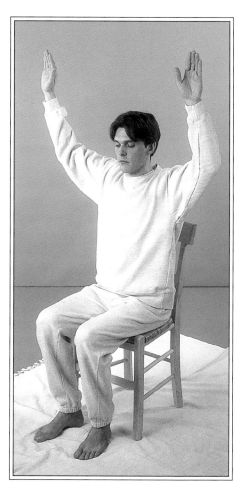

YOGA IS A RELATIONSHIP

The above principles link together to offer possibilities that enhance your relationship with yourself through your practice. This opens the possibility that a deepening of your practice comes not from adding more difficult postures but from refining your relationship with what you already have. Life is already full of pressures to go for the newest model, to bring more in from the outside rather than concentrating on bringing more out from the inside. So you need to take care that you do not become an avid consumer of a new posture or new technique purely for the sake of it.

Yoga is a relationship within which you commit yourself to depth of involvement rather than breadth of involvement. In that sense, yoga is no different from how any relationship with someone or something you care for and wish to spend time with should be. From this relationship you can eventually start to experience the fruits that arise from the time, care, work and attention. Keep the following words of a teacher from long ago in your mind as you adapt yoga to suit your particular needs:

"Yoga is known through practice.
Practice itself leads to Yoga. One who cares for their practice for a long time tastes the fruits."

PRACTICE 1

A simple practice sequence follows which aims at reducing stress generally, and in particular tension headaches which often accompany it. The practice uses postures with breathing techniques and a simple visualization and is helpful where the emphasis is on generally relaxing and lessening accumulated stress.

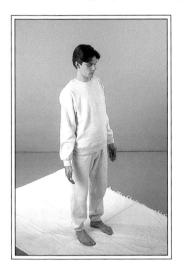

1 Standing with your feet slightly apart, allow your body to settle. Focus on deepening your breathing. When it is full and steady, raise your arms as you breathe in.

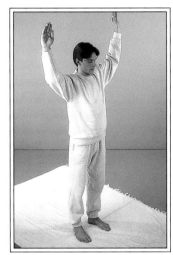

2 The speed of this movement is decided by your breath. Finish the inhale with your arms above your head, shoulders relaxed. Bring your arms down as you breathe out. Repeat eight times.

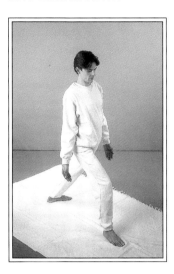

1 Stand with your feet about 60–90cm (2–3ft) apart with the back foot at an angle and the leg straight. As you breathe in, raise your arms while pushing the front knee forwards with the back leg braced.

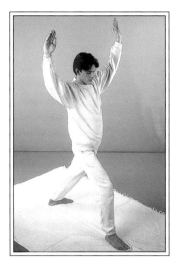

2 Complete the inhale with your arms raised and your chest open. Wait a few seconds, then start to breathe out, lowering the arms and straightening the front leg. Repeat this sequence eight times.

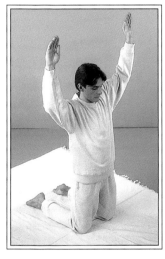

1 Kneel up with your legs slightly apart and your feet relaxed. As you breathe in, raise your arms, keeping the shoulders loose and your chest open. As you breathe out, bend forward, keeping your back rounded.

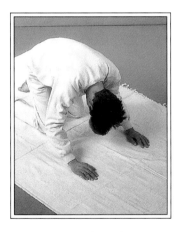

2 Continue to breathe out until your hands are on the ground and your shoulders relaxed. Wait a few seconds then breathe in while lifting your arms and then your back. Repeat eight times.

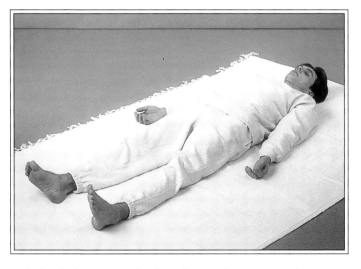

3 To finish, lie on your back with your feet apart and your arms slightly away from your sides. Allow your breathing to settle and then slow it down while softening your body, as if you were melting into the floor. Relax in this position for about two to three minutes.

The second practice sequence concentrates on alleviating the symptoms of accumulative stress which might occur after many hours working at a keyboard or computer screen. This practice serves both as a curative of aches and pains, and as a preventive to help in minimizing any build-up of tension in the head, neck and shoulder areas.

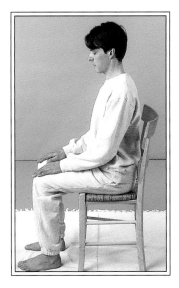

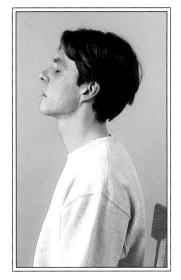

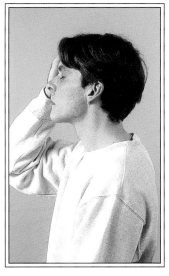

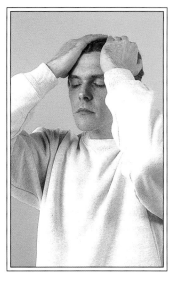

1 Sit on a chair with your feet apart and your spine erect. Rest your hands on your thighs. Keeping your eyes closed, imagine that you are focusing on a point on the floor in front of you. Maintain this internal focus for a few minutes, breathing gently, before relaxing.

2 As you slowly breathe in, gently and slowly raise your head while keeping your shoulders relaxed. As you breathe out, again gently and slowly, lower your head without allowing your back to slump. Repeat this movement eight times.

3 From the same sitting position, slowly breathe in and raise one hand to touch your forehead, while at the same time raising your head. As you breathe out, lower your hand and head. Repeat eight times, alternating hands.

4 This time, raise both hands at the same time as you breathe in and lower both as you breathe out. Repeat this sequence eight times.

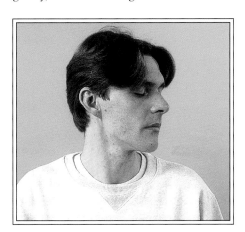

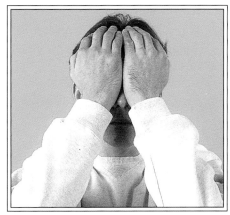

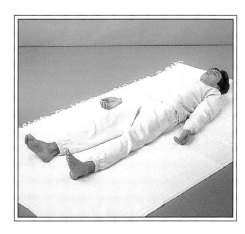

5 Now rest your hands on your thighs while you turn your head from side to side with each breath. As you breathe out, slowly turn your head to the left; as you breathe in, bring your head back to the centre, repeat to the right. Repeat this sequence eight times.

6 Still with your hands on your thighs, take a breath. As you breathe out, raise your hands, bringing your palms over your eyes. Breathe once, then as you breathe in again return your hands to your thighs. Repeat four times.

7 Lie on the floor, let your breathing settle and your body soften. Focus your attention on any tightness in your body and use your exhale to release it. After two minutes, rest for a minute or so.

FINAL THOUGHTS

Some of the possibilities that underpin yoga through practice have been introduced above. The practice of yoga as power, meditation and therapy has been considered. Each aspect, although having its own approach and focus, complements and offers the practitioner a holistic model for the development of body, mind and well-being.

In the West today therapy is the starting point that most often brings people to yoga. The use of yoga as therapy has been approached from the viewpoint of the person rather than the problem. It is not appropriate in considering yoga practice to "lump" people together as back-pain sufferers or migraine sufferers. It is true to say there are some common characteristics within various problems, but then so there are in all areas of people's lives. People live together in groups determined by commonalities and yet each person is unique. This is what needs to be considered when proposing practices for individuals: "Teach what is inside you, not as it applies to you yourself but as it applies to the other."

With this as a priority, some basic principles common for anybody wishing to practice yoga were considered. Such concepts offer an intelligent means to enter into the spirit of the practice with the least disturbance to what is, in the field of therapy, already an unhealthy body and mind. These principles are also offered as a way to deepen your relationship with yoga. Through that link you will discover something new about yourselves. From the view of yoga, this means that the way things affect you can change and you can influence the process of change and its consequences. From here, two different practices, designed to support two students who, confronted with the same problem, turned out to have very different needs, were proposed.

RIGHT: Practise a little yoga every day for the best benefits.

FURTHER PRACTICE

If you wish to take your interest in yoga further, take lessons with a qualified yoga teacher, choosing one who concentrates on your particular interest. You should do a little each day rather than practise irregularly. Wear loose or stretchy clothing when practising and use a mat or folded blanket on the floor. Don't practise yoga with a full bladder or bowels, and wait at least three hours after a heavy meal. Take a shower after a practice session to complete the relaxation and refreshment.

Yoga is a journey to be experienced. However, that journey not only requires patience and perseverance, but also enthusiasm and confidence. In this respect, as in any relationship between people, it is necessary to consider priorities. To students interested in undertaking a home practice, two suggestions are offered.

First, think of yoga as a new book. Before you try to fit this book into what is probably an overcrowded bookshelf, take a decision to remove an existing book to make room for the new one. Do not, however, try to remove a large book and make unrealistic adjustments in the space on your shelf. Instead, take out a slim volume and this way, create realistic space without yoga becoming another pressure.

This leads on to the second suggestion. Life is often divided into agendas, two of which are headed "chore" and "reward". Try to keep some room on the latter list for your practice in the same way that you would greet an old friend. Take time in their company and return to your everyday life rejuvenated and better able to embrace your surroundings.

MOXIBUSTION

The practice of acupuncture has become quite widespread in the West, and indeed throughout the world in the past 25 years or so. Most people are aware that it is an ancient Chinese system of healing that involves the use of fine needles inserted into the body at specific points to achieve a particular therapeutic effect. Acupuncture has a long lineage; indeed, many of the principles of diagnosis and treatment were laid down in the *Huangdi Neijing* (or *Yellow Emperor's Canon of Medicine*) – the earliest Chinese medical text extant, dating from 500–300 BC. The origins of acupuncture probably go back much further.

Acupuncture's underlying principle is that of vital force (or *qi*) animating mind and body. For various complex reasons the flow and distribution of *qi* can become unbalanced or out of harmony, and the aim of acupuncture is to determine the pattern and underlying causes of this disharmony and rectify it by needling particular points on the body.

Less well-known than acupuncture is moxibustion, an integral part of Chinese medicine and most commonly practised in conjunction with acupuncture. In moxibustion, a small quantity of the moxa herb (or mugwort – *Artemisia vulgaris*) is burned on the end of an acupuncture needle (while the needle is in position) or in the form of a small stick or cone placed directly on the skin (usually being removed

BELOW: Acupuncture needles, moxibustion sticks and the moxa herb are all used in the practice of moxibustion.

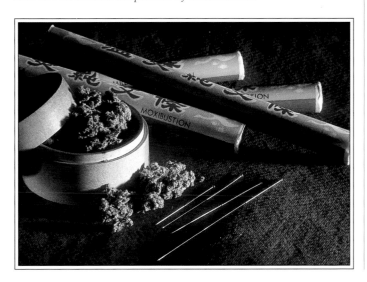

RIGHT: The meridian lines used in both acupuncture and moxibustion.

before the skin is burned). Moxa can be used in its own right or to augment the effect of the needles; its use is indicated where the body's energies need warming or tonifying, or to help move stagnation of the *qi*.

The use of needles for self-treatment is clearly inappropriate but the use of moxa in the form of the moxa stick can be very effective in the area of health promotion and maintenance. In particular, it is useful for its general tonic effect, especially for the middle-aged or elderly. Its application can be wonderfully soothing and relaxing for mind and body, and this alone is of great benefit to health in general.

There are, however, some contraindications for the use of moxa:

❧ During pregnancy.

❧ With people with hypertension (high blood pressure).

❧ On any rashes, especially if the skin is broken.

❧ During acute illness in general but in particular if this involves feeling heat or fullness anywhere in the body, a raised temperature or any inflammation.

❧ In cases where the inhalation of smoke is an irritant (the moxa stick gives off herbal-smelling smoke).

❧ On any sensitive part of the body such as the face.

A few people may not enjoy sessions involving the use of moxa or respond well afterwards. There may be a number of reasons for this: for example, their energy may already be "over-heated". As a general rule, it is best not to use moxa again if any symptoms seem worse after its use.

HOW TO USE THE MOXA STICK

For mild moxibustion the moxa stick provides the most convenient means for self-application. About an inch or so of the stick will be used in any one session.

The stick is best lit from a candle; this takes about half a minute and it is helpful to blow on the lighted end occasionally to improve combustion. It is also quite useful to remove about 2.5 cm (1 in) of the outer layer of paper (but *not* the inner layer), since this helps the stick to burn more evenly. During a session, the ash will occasionally have to be tapped off into an ashtray. While burning, the stick imparts rather a strong-smelling herbal smoke, which is quite pleasant, but some ventilation is recommended.

After a session, it is essential to ensure that the stick is properly extinguished. It is rarely sufficient merely to "stub" the lighted end out – it tends to start burning again. The best way is to cut off the lighted end with a sharp knife, then dampen the end, being careful, of course, not to get water on to the unburned section of the stick, which should then be stored in a dry place for further use.

APPLICATION OF THE MOXA STICK

The application of moxa should be a very relaxing and pleasurable experience; you should stop if it does not feel so. The sensation of warmth emanating from the stick on to the skin should not be so great as to be uncomfortable. The distance that the stick is held from the skin will vary from person to person and from point to point. About 2.5cm (1in) from the skin is a rough average. As the stick is held near the skin, the sensation of warmth will gradually increase; the stick is pulled away before the sensation of heat becomes uncomfortable and after a few seconds the stick can be brought nearer the skin again. This "dabbing" action backwards and forwards with the stick is repeated a number of times, until the skin feels hot and slightly pink and the sensation of warmth feels as if it has penetrated the body. Another easier and perhaps more relaxing method of using the stick is to find a distance from the skin that allows the sensation of warmth to build up to a comfortable level that can be maintained for a period of time without having to "dab" the stick.

There is no fixed rule as to how long to spend using the moxa stick during a session. The session should last as long as it takes to allow the selected point or points to become quite warm, and the skin slightly pink with the feeling that the heat has penetrated. On average, this might be about a minute or two for each point, but sometimes longer. If all the points mentioned in the step sequence were used together, the session should take about 10–20 minutes. It is very important not to overheat a point as there is a very slight chance this might lead to the skin blistering after the session. This will not happen if the application is gentle.

The number of sessions or their frequency can also vary. It is recommended, however, that the sessions should not be more than twice weekly, with breaks of one or two weeks every month or so. There is no advantage in using moxa over an indefinite period and it is desirable to have regular breaks. Provided the sessions feel pleasant, relaxing and beneficial, many of the points mentioned here can be regularly warmed with moxa for a limited period. Be aware of the contraindications, however.

HOW TO USE THE MOXA STICK

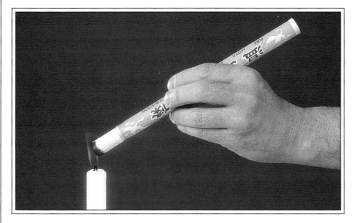

1 Light the moxa stick with a candle, holding the tip in the flame until it is smoking steadily. Blow on the lighted end to encourage combustion.

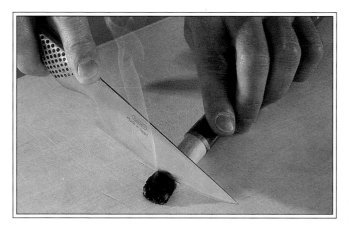

2 When you have finished the session, cut off the lighted end of the moxa stick with a sharp knife on to a board. Make sure it is completely cooled before you store it.

SOME RECOMMENDED POINTS

Some points which are suitable for you to practise at home are illustrated here. Remember to take care not to hold sticks for more than a minute or two at a time over each point. Keep asking your partner if they are comfortable: they should feel a pleasant warmth and no more. Before you apply the stick, draw small circles on the correct points of the body with a pen to ensure that you will focus it on the right spot.

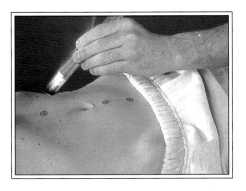

1 Stomach 36 (*zusanli* – "leg three miles"). You will find this point just underneath the knee.

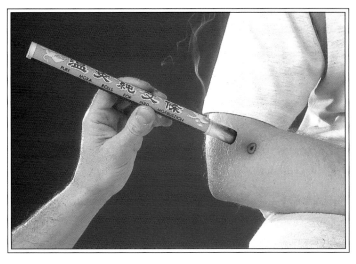

2 Large Intestine 10 (*shousanli* – "arm three miles"). This point is located just above the elbow joint.

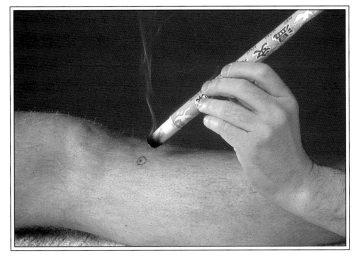

3 Directing Vessel Points: REN 4, the first of three points located on the stomach, just below the ribs.

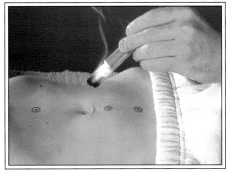

4 REN 6, the second stomach point is found just below the navel.

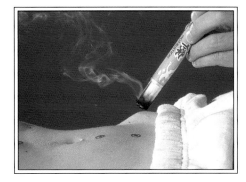

5 REN 8 is found halfway between the navel and the pubic bone.

6 Using the moxa stick on areas of the body is one of the most effective uses for mild moxibustion. It is appropriate for areas which feel chronically cold, weak, stiff or achy, including joints. It is not generally recommended in cases of acute pain. To apply, simply hold the moxa stick above a general area of the body – for example the lower back – for a few seconds for a general feeling of warmth and well-being.

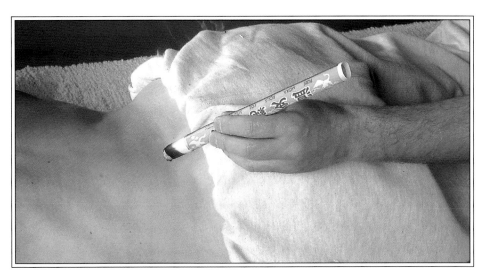

USEFUL ADDRESSES

UK

AROMATHERAPY
International Society of Professional
Aromatherapists
The Hinckley and District Hospital
Mount Road
Hinckley
Leicestershire LE10 1AG

International Federation of
Aromatherapists
4 Eastmearn Road
London SE21 8HA

HERBALISM
National Institute of Medical Herbalists
56 Longbrook Street
Exeter
Devon EX4 6AH

The Herb Society
134 Buckingham Palace Road
London SW1W 9SA

HOMEOPATHY
The Homeopathic Society
2 Powis Place
Great Ormond Steet
London WC1N 3HT

BACH FLOWER REMEDIES
Dr Edward Bach Centre
Mount Vernon Sotwell
Wallingford
Oxon OX10 0PZ

HYPNOTHERAPY
International Association of Hypno-
analysts
The Institute of Complementary
Medicine PO Box 194

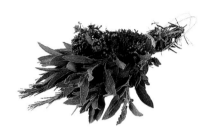

London SE16 1QZ (write with SAE)
Tel: (01202) 316496

MOXIBUSTION
AcuMedic
101-105 Camden High Street
London NW1 7JN (suppliers of sticks)

MEDITATION
Gateway Books
The Hollies
Wellow
Bath BA2 8QJ (for books and tapes)

US

ASSOCIATIONS
American Association of Naturopathic
Physicians (AANP)
2366 Eastlake Avenue
Suite 322
Seattle, WA 98102

American Chiropractic Association
1701 Clarendon Blvd
Arlington, VA 22209

American Osteopathic Association
142 East Ontario Street
Chicago, IL 60611

College of Maharishi Ayur-Veda
Health Center
PO Box 282
Fairfield, IA 52556

HERB SUPPLIERS
Seeds Blum
Idaho City State
Boise, ID 83706

HYPNOTHERAPY
American Society of Clinical Hypnosis
2200 E. Devon Ave., Suite 291
Des Plaines, IL 60018

AUSTRALIA

AROMATHERAPY
International Federation of
Aromatherapists
National Inf. Line: 190 2240 125

HERBALISM
National Herbalist Association
PO Box 61
Broadway, NSW 2069

HOMEOPATHY
Australian Institute of Homeopathy
PO Box 122
Roseville NSW 2069

Bach Flower Shop
309 Little Collins Street
Melbourne Vic 3000

Brauer Biotherapies Pty Ltd
1 Para Road
Tanunda, SA 5352

Fitch's Pharmacy
731 Hay Street
Perth WA 9000

INDEX

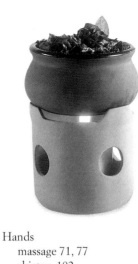

Abdomen
    exercises 41
    massage 77
Acupuncture 88, 124
Alexander technique 87
Arms
    exercises 41
    massage 72, 77
    shiatsu 102
Aromatherapy
    air, oils in 23
    essential therapies 22
    massage oils 25
    oils 22
    water, oils in 24
Autogenics 62, 63

Bach flower remedies 26
Back
    massage 75
    shiatsu 104
Bodywork 66

Carbohydrates 32
Chiropractic 84
Cranio-sacral therapy 85

Diet
    exercise, and 30, 31
    healthy eating 36
    medicine, and 8
    week's eating programme 37

Ears, shiatsu 101
Eastern approaches 88
Exercise
    arm and abdomen exercises 41
    bending and squatting 42
    diet, and 30, 31
    effect of 38
    floor exercises 43
    recommended 38
    shoulder and neck exercises
        40
    warming up 39

Face
    massage 70, 78
    shiatsu 99, 100
Fats 34
Feet
    massage 82, 83
    reflexology 80, 81
    shiatsu 105, 106

Hands
    massage 71, 77
    shiatsu, 102
Head
    cranio-sacral therapy 85
    shiatsu 98
Healing 64, 65
Herb teas 16, 17
Herbal medicine 10, 11
Herbs
    aromatic seeds 13
    drying 10
    food, in 12
    leafy 12
    supplements 18
Homeopathy 27
Hydrotherapy 44
Hypnotherapy 48
    self-hypnotic induction 49

Iridology 45

Legs
    massage 73, 76
    shiatsu 105, 106
Life force 91

Makko Ho exercises
    bladder and kidneys 111
    breathing 108
    heart and small intestine 110
    liver and gall bladder 112
    lungs and large intestine 110
    practice 109
    triple heater and heart
        protector 111
Massage
    abdomen 77
    arms 72, 77
    back 75
    face 70, 78

foot 82, 83
hands 71, 77
legs 73, 76
neck 72
partner, with 74-78, 82, 83
preventive 70
professional 66
self 66, 70-73
shoulders 70
Meditation 88
    body, for 54, 55
    focusing 59
    mind, for 56
    periods of 57, 58
    posture 58
    practising 57, 58
    schools of 54
    yoga 114
Minerals 35
Moxibustion
    moxa stick, use and
        application of 125
    principle 124
    recommended points 126

Naturopathy 28
Neck
    exercises 40
    massage 72
    shiatsu 99

Osteopathy 86

Plants, medicines from 8
Proteins 33
Psychotherapy 60, 61

Reflexology 80, 81
Rolfing 79
Roots 15

Self-hypnotic induction 49
    affirmations 52
    calm technique 51
    haven 51
    physical relaxation 49
    stairs, imagining 50
    swish technique 53
    visualization 52
Shiatsu
    back 104
    chest and abdomen 103
    ears 101
    effects, 95

face 99, 100
hands 102
head 98
history and philosophy 91
ki 91
legs and feet 105, 106
meaning 90
meridian stimulation 98-107
meridian system 93
neck 99
organs, table of 92
partner, with 96, 97
practitioner, with 94
prone position 97
qi 90, 91
sessions 95
shoulders and arms 102
touch, importance of 90
Shoulders
    exercises 40
    massage 70
    shiatsu 102
Stress management 46, 49-53

Vitamins 35

Yoga
    appropriate asanas, choosing
        116
    breathing, 118
    mediation, as 114
    movement 117
    person, adapting posture to
        119
    power, as 114
    practice sequences 121, 122
    practices 115
    principles 120, 123
    relationship, as 120

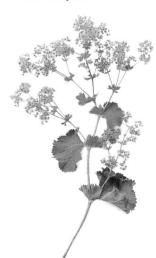